Prepublication Quotes

*"I thoroughly enjoyed reading **For Women Only**, just as I felt reading **Parts Psychology**. I really like your method of teaching by case example."*
—Louis Tinnin, M.D., Emeritus Professor, West Virginia University; Founder, Intensive Trauma Institute

"[This] book will make a positive difference for many women and their families."
—Rev. Barbara Louw, Traumatologist, Pretoria, South Africa.

"I enjoyed reading this excellent case study."
—Gavin Williams, M.A., M.Phil., London, UK

"It is a great, great book!! I found it both a fascinating story, as well as clinically enlightening. The subject matter is unique, and I love the approach."
—Monica Rubinow Tenner, Developmental Trauma and Attachment Therapist, Pasadena, California.

"I really enjoyed reading this. The book has a good clear style, flows well. Will the publisher allow me to translate it into Portuguese and Spanish?"
—Esly Regina de Carvalho, PhD, EMDR Psychotherapy for Adults in Brasília, Brazil.

For Women Only, Book 1

For Women Only, Book 1

Healing Childbirth PTSD and Postpartum Depression with Parts Psychology

With an Excerpt of Chapter 1 from *Parts Psychology*

By

Jay Noricks PhD

New University Press LLC

www.newuniversitypress.com

Los Angeles • Las Vegas

Part 2

Excerpt:

*Parts Psychology: A Trauma-Based, Self-State
Therapy for Emotional Healing*

Preface

For Women Only, Book 1 is not really for women only. However, it is the first in a series of books intended to address women's issues in a new way. Specifically, the series will take a Parts Psychology perspective of examining problems as they are experienced through a person's parts, self-states, subpersonalities, sides or ego states. All of these terms are interchangeable labels for the multiple ways in which people—normal and abnormal—present themselves to others.

The first audience for this little book is the community of psychotherapists and counselors that is always looking for new ways to help their patients. My hope is that other therapists will find something useful here for their own practices. Doing work within the paradigm of Parts Psychology requires a major shift in how the mind is understood. In particular, the therapist must recognize that the mind is not unitary. It is naturally multiple: divided into parts that normally but not always work seamlessly together. When someone is wounded to the degree that they cannot get a painful experience out of their mind, deeper work than the standard talk therapy is necessary for healing. Healing requires locating the wounded part of the self and treating it directly. This book provides an introduction to doing that deeper work.

The second intended audience is a more general one. I have written with a minimum of technical terms with an eye toward making the narrative easily followed by the average college freshman. My hope is that word will spread that healing is available for both the wounds of ordinary life and those of more dramatic lived experiences.

A large number of society's members find themselves suffering from unnecessary trauma and trauma-like experiences that continue to haunt them. Some of these experiences originate in childhood. Some have a more recent origin: in work, in relationships, or in normal but painful life events, such as death, divorce, and illness. Most people are not aware that their emotional pain can be completely healed. This book aims to illustrate this healing.

Acknowledgements

Each of the following colleagues made helpful remarks on one or another draft of this book. I am
grateful to each of them for taking the time out of
their busy schedules to read and criticize my earlier
drafts. Sometimes I took their advice and sometimes I
chose otherwise, but I always read carefully what they
had to say:

Daniel Berarduchi, James Brittain, Chad
Broderick, Jerri Gallegos-Carr, Esly Regina de
Carvalho, Linda C. Chambers, Robin Dilley,
Kelly Halvorsen, Barbara Louw, Chenee Marx,
Oraine Ramoo, Patrick R. Scott, Monica Rubinow Tenner, Louis Tinnin, Gavin Williams. I
am especially indebted to, Jonathan Pishner,
from whose close editing and provocative
questions I benefited greatly.

Of course, all errors and difficulties in communicating
are exclusively mine.

Chapter 1
Introduction

Catherine called me from Denver one morning to schedule an appointment on her next visit to Las Vegas, the home base for my clinic. Maria, Catherine's psychotherapist neighbor, had referred her to me. Maria had taken my workshop in Parts Psychology in Denver during the previous year and believed that Catherine could benefit from the visualization work the workshop emphasized. The workshop trains therapists to work with patients' internal *parts* or *self-states* to heal traumatic and trauma-like events. Maria thought that this approach might be exactly what Catherine needed to heal from the painful experiences associated with her pregnancy and the 36 hours of labor she endured before giving birth to her son.

As the district sales manager for her nationwide company at the relatively young age of 34, Catherine had considerable flexibility in arranging her travel plans. She would fly to Las Vegas for one-hour sessions on consecutive days every two weeks. In all, we met for six sessions spread over six weeks. This is a relatively small number of sessions for healing major issues, but I originally thought we could do the work in even less time, just three sessions. However, I revised that estimate quickly after beginning therapy with Catherine. It was soon apparent that Catherine met the criteria for posttraumatic stress disorder (PTSD) as well as postpartum depression. This was not surprising but, based upon our early phone and email exchanges, I did not expect the added complexity. Still, these diagnoses made no difference in the way we did the therapy. In fact, despite the severity of symptoms, the therapy was fairly routine. Consequently, Catherine's story seemed ideal for illustrating how Parts Psychology works with stand-alone trauma (as opposed to chronic traumatic exposure).

Our first session provided strong hints that more than three sessions might be necessary to process the trauma. The first indication was the depression screen Catherine filled out and brought to the meeting. Her responses to the questionnaire suggested depression in the moderate to severe range. She seemed unaware that she had been experiencing postpartum depression since the birth of her child eight months previously. Her physical appearance also hinted that she was experiencing emotional difficulties. When I first met her in the waiting room, she sat hunched over and seemed to draw her shoulders forward to enclose her chest, squeezing herself into a smaller space. Her blond hair was long, reaching her shoulders, but at that time was hidden underneath her shirt and a Denver Broncos cap pulled low over her eyes. Her smile seemed forced as she looked up without fully raising her head.

The next indication of complexity appeared in the story she narrated in that first session. Her mother, whom she described as her life-long best friend, had inexplicably abandoned Catherine in an emotional sense when she learned of the pregnancy. On the basis of what Catherine revealed in the narrative, I silently hypothesized that this abandonment might have had a significant effect on both the difficulty of the childbirth and the depression that followed.

The following pages describe Catherine's six sessions of therapy. When we began, she met criteria for both PTSD and postpartum depression. At the end of our work, she met criteria for neither. Her 18 months of painful experiences had transformed into a personal history of insight and wisdom, a history that was no longer painful.

The next section contains a narrative of our first session. The story Catherine told served as our touchstone. It provided the information about Catherine's experiences that guided our work in the five later sessions. We would return to it throughout the therapy in order to assess Catherine's progress. The protocol for collecting the narrative is straightforward:

1. Establish the normal pre-trauma context.

2. Elicit the story of the trauma.

3. Return the story to a new normal context.

4. Note the emotions and tensions shown by the patient during the narrative.

Ideally, the narrative serves to alert the therapist to the high-energy, emotionally powerful moments in the patient's story. These moments are revisited in the ongoing therapy. Additionally, the narrative format of moving from normal life through traumatic events to new normal life aims to reduce the sharp distinction between traumatic and non-traumatic experiences. The format intends to aid the patient in developing the view that her story is a factual history of her life and not a story of continuing pain. As history, her story is situated in the past.

Chapter 2
Session 1: The Narrative

Catherine's story is presented in her own words, mostly as they were spoken, drawn from my hand-written notes. Inevitably, I have left out a few phrases here and there, but the text is otherwise true to both our recollections. I did not want to intrude into the sessions with the use of a tape recorder. My occasional remarks are presented in brackets and generally record Catherine's nonverbal expressions. Additionally, I sometimes use brackets to indicate some of my own thoughts during the narrative.

"I have always been driven to succeed, to excel. I finished college in four years and began a career. I returned to graduate school and was the first in my class to finish and get approval for my thesis. I went from sales leader in my office to managing another branch to becoming a district manager. I was established in my career and so was my husband.

"We decided now was the time to have a child, maybe two. My company made it easy to have children and keep your career. I got pregnant within two weeks. We were at Disneyworld on vacation and I noticed that my body wasn't feeling good—I missed my cycle. I tested positive. When we knew for sure I told my parents.

"My father was happy; he hugged me. But my mother was not so happy. She didn't smile even. All she said was a sarcastic 'You timed that perfectly!' I didn't understand what she meant. All I could think of was that she meant that I chose to have a baby when *I* was ready and not when *she* was. She wasn't happy for me. We used to do everything together; talked every day at least once. We were best friends. Later, at a lunch, she was critical of me and bossy. I didn't like that. I told her I needed to have low stress while I was pregnant. She got angry and said she would talk to me any way she wanted! After this lunch, we didn't talk. [Tears, difficulty speaking.] I tried to reconnect with her but she was absent through the pregnancy.

"I enjoyed my pregnancy throughout. I did everything I could to do a perfect natural childbirth. I took classes, exercised, did yoga, took all the right vitamins, everything. I had an induced pregnancy one week past my due date because my doctor had to be out of town the week after that and I was afraid I'd have the baby before he came back. I had all my plans in place so there wouldn't be any problems.

"I went into labor but didn't know it. I had contractions but the nurses had to show me I had them. No one told me how difficult it would be! [Tears.] I had no clue how painful it would be! I was feeling the pain after 12 hours. After 15 hours, I went to the water tub—I wanted to do birth in the water tub—that's when the pain got even worse. [Tears.] I finally gave in to the epidural, but it didn't take away the pain. The anesthesiologist even tried different brands but it didn't work. It felt like I was in a huge ocean on fire and being hit in the back with huge waves [of pain].

"I kept at a dilation of five [centimeters] for hours and hours, but there was hardly any movement. [Tears.] By the 34th or 35th hour, I was thinking of a C-section. I was exhausted. I gave in and asked for it. But they all said 'keep going, almost there!'—the water broke at the 35th hour—things began to speed up. It was time to push but I didn't know what that meant. I used a visualization of my pregnant self to push the baby out. [Imagery noted.] The baby was finally out—not breathing at first! But he was okay! I did not feel happy—I was shaking, seeing double, and unable to speak for what seemed like two hours. [Tears.] I felt invaded by the doctor. The nurses were pushing out the remaining fluids. They couldn't give me the baby because they had to be sure he was okay. It was 36 hours! They took me to postpartum—I can't remember two hours—I remember the next day, breast feeding—I didn't know how—it was so hard! [Tears, strong emotion.] I had so many different emotions. I kept telling the baby he was doing good: 'Good job!' My body was in a lot of pain afterwards—back pain—it took forever to get out of the bed to go to the bathroom. The baby took so long to feed—one half hour a side, nipping, nibbling. He would fall asleep and then nurse and fall asleep again. And then I had to chart the feeding times every two hours. I was so tired!

"My mom and dad came the next day. I was surprised that my mother was there. She took a video of us. I was there four days. I felt alone. Just my husband and me. Finally I went home. I was so tired! My parents came the next day but my mother didn't help. She only helped me two times with the baby's bath. They live in walking distance!"

We were nearing the end of the session and I wanted Catherine to complete the trauma narrative and move on in her story to a new normal—a description of her life now that it had normalized again. Thus, I asked her to skip three months into the future.

"My husband went back to his regular work routine—80 hours or more of work per week. I was alone most of the first two months—we tried to find a nanny—that was a nightmare! [Strong emotion.] In the third month he finally learned how to help with the baby, though he still worked 60 to 70 hours a week. He slowly cut back on his work hours. In the third month, I thought momentarily that I could have another baby—then, *no!* From then until now [at eight months postpartum], *no way!*"

Still trying to help Catherine connect to a new normal context, I asked her to skip another four months and imagine the future when her baby would be 12 months old.

"He's crawling already. At 12 months he'll be walking and not breast feeding. I want it to be better by 12 months. I don't love the baby state but he's cute and makes me laugh."

This ended our first session. We began with a normal pre-trauma context, focused upon the details of the trauma narrative, and tried to connect to a new normal state. Unfortunately, Catherine's lingering postpartum depression prevented a smooth narrative transition to a new normal. That is, she had not yet experienced the transition into a life without emotional pain. She had not returned to whatever she would view as *normal* life.

At the end of each session, I made it a point to note how I thought the next session might go. We could always adjust our focus, depending upon Catherine's thoughts and feelings at the beginning of the next session. However, I wanted to have a general plan in place as a framework for continued work. In this case, I thought we would probably aim to reduce the pain and exhaustion still seemingly attached to Catherine's traumatic memories. Alternatively, we might work on issues involving her mother because the narrative suggested significant attachment wounds that affected the trauma of the birth process. Catherine's issues with her mother, it seemed to me, might have affected both the difficulty of childbirth and her postpartum depression.

I will return to Catherine's therapy, including the relationship with her mother, following an introduction to the more important elements of the theory of internal parts (self-states) and how to heal them. Healing parts of the self is the primary means of healing the whole patient in this paradigm. A more in-depth description of the theory appears in my book *Parts Psychology*.

Chapter 3
Parts Psychology

Parts Psychology is the trauma-based theoretical framework within which I work.[1] The basic premise is that almost all mental health issues derive from earlier life experiences, most of which can be described as traumatic or trauma-like in their intensity. What this means for therapy is that therapist and patient work together to discover the early experiences that are the foundation for the patient's problems. Normally, that would mean some exploration of the patient's childhood and teen years in search of at least some of the sources of current-time issues.

In Catherine's case, that work was unnecessary because the sources of her problems were largely self-evident in the narrative of the first session. Her childbirth was traumatic and she had lost the positive connection (attachment bond) with her mother that she had enjoyed all of her life. Consequently, we could start work immediately on the trauma and loss.

For patients with less obvious trauma and attachment wounds, the therapy involves more systematic work to locate the relevant memories. The Parts Psychology framework holds that these memories are stored within subdivisions of the larger self called *parts* or *self-states*. A part is not just a container for autobiographical memories but is also an agent of thought and action. A part has a submind that blends or retracts from the core self, depending upon the environment. Thus, we get such thinking as "A part of me knows I should kick him out, but a part of me loves him and cannot imagine life without him." Each of these "parts" provides a different way of thinking and a different course of action for the person.

The healing of a patient results from the healing of the part of the patient that carries the problem memories. The patient is automatically healed when the part is healed. This is so because, for a particular issue, the part and the patient are the same. They act as one.

The therapist and the patient work together to resolve the relevant painful memories. The resolution of these memories results from permanently releasing (i.e., neutralizing) the negative emotions and sensations attached to the patient's difficult autobiographical memories. Following this processing, patients retain the knowledge and insight that these memories bring but they permanently release the emotional pain. (In some cases, positively experienced memories must also be neutralized—for example, the romantic feelings toward a lost love that interfere with a patient's attachment to a new spouse. However, in Catherine's case, we were concerned only with negatively experienced memories.)

The approach draws upon some of the important ideas found in other theories, especially those theories that emphasize the normal multiplicity of the mind. The best examples of these theories are John and Helen Watkins's *Ego State* therapy; Richard C. Schwartz's *Internal Family Systems* therapy; Hal and Sidra Stone's *Voice Dialog;* John Rowan's work with subpersonalities; and Roberto Assagioli's *Psychosynthesis.*[2] In all of these approaches the therapist works with internal self-states, variously called parts, *subpersonalities, sides, ego states,* and *voices.*

The normal multiplicity of mind is not a new idea. Morton Prince, one of the founders of American psychology, described the presence of normal subpersonalities (he called them "sides") as early as 1925.[3] Internal self-states, surprisingly for most people, have minds of their own. They have their own agendas, their own senses of self, usually their own self-images, and most importantly, a continuing desire to exist.

For those not familiar with the concept of internal parts with a life of their own, I include a short introduction below that introduces their presence in everyday life. It is the same introduction I provide to most of my patients at our first session.

Introduction to Parts

If you are a parent, think about how you feel, or used to feel, when you were tending to hungry, fussy, or needy children. If you haven't tended to children, think about any experience that demanded a lot of attention from you when you had too many things to do. Or, think about how you feel in a demanding work setting or any social situation where you feel unappreciated or undervalued. Then, switch your focus and think about how you feel, or remember feeling, on an exciting romantic date. Take a moment to compare these different ways of feeling. These feeling states can be so different that you might almost feel that you are two different people. When you think about how you can experience life so differently in different situations, you are recognizing some of the parts that make up your whole personality.

Parts Psychology is based upon the idea that it is normal for us to have many different ways of being ourselves. But some of these ways of being ourselves could use some help in therapy. Each of these ways of being forms a part, or self-state, within our minds. One part is dominant when we are sad and another part is dominant when we are angry. Actually, there is sometimes a cluster of parts or self-states that present as sad or mad, but for simplicity I will talk about single states. At any given moment, a single dominant part largely determines how we act. When challenged, for example, we might react with anxiety, anger, or even with calm assurance, but we cannot act with all three of these emotional states at the same time. The set of beliefs, attitudes, and feelings that dominate our response to the challenge is what I am calling a part or self-state.

The idea of parts is common in everyday language. For example, "A part of me wants to tell my boss to go to hell, but another part of me says I should mellow out because I need this job." Sometimes we compare a rational view to an emotional one: "My brain tells me to do one thing but my heart tells me something else." Heart and brain here are the same as parts. If you think for a moment about the way you feel when you take one point of view or the other, you can easily recognize how different these parts of you are.

These are the parts with which the parts psychologist helps you work. Especially when the parts are extreme in their effect on you, you probably cannot permanently heal yourself without working with these parts. Examples include problems with rage, extended grief, panic attacks, behavioral addictions, and unwanted romantic feelings. And there are many more. In fact, every problem that brings you to therapy can be helped by working with the parts of you that are wounded in some way.

A part is an internal entity or structure with its own way of thinking and feeling. In short, it has its own submind. It has its own way of viewing the world and its own agenda. The highest priority for any given part of you is to help you. Even an extremely critical part of you that seems to want to destroy you aims to help you. It's just trying too hard.

The most important content of a part or self-state is a set of memories of events where the part was present. A romantic part has a different set of memories from a harassed mom or dad part. Healing your problems requires that we work with the memories of the part of you that carries the problem. If the problem is work stress, for example, we probably do not need to work with the romantic part of you.

The memories we work with could be as recent as last night's argument with your spouse, or they may be ancient memories of your fear as a child when Mom and Dad were arguing and threatening divorce. A part of you recorded those memories and stored them, sometimes in places where you cannot easily reach them. Sometimes you may not even remember an experience until we work with the part of you that contains the memories. But the memories do not disappear, and they don't heal without help. They continue to affect you in the present. In doing therapy with parts, our job is to neutralize (heal) those memories so that they are no longer triggered by present-time experience. You will keep the memories and the knowledge that goes with them, but you will learn to let go of the painful emotions attached to them.

Your therapist will help you visualize the parts of you that present problems in your life. But you may want to do some experimenting on your own. One way to recognize one of your own parts is to think about someone you really dislike. Hold a picture of that person in your mind for a moment and check to see if just thinking of this person causes you to feel a strong emotion or sensation. If so, you can simply direct your thoughts to that emotion or sensation and ask it to give you an image of itself in your mind. This simple request allows about 50 percent of patients to immediately produce an internal image of the part of them that feels the strong emotion.

Other techniques will allow nearly all other patients to produce an internal image. The kind of image that pops up most often is simply an image of yourself at a different age in your life or with a different facial expression or body attitude. In Catherine's case there was a part that looked like her when she was aged 22.

It is also normal for other kinds of images to represent the part you are looking for. The color red or a ball of fire, for example, is a common image we use to represent anger. Clouds or grey veils are images we sometimes use to represent the depressed part of ourselves. Sometimes a cartoon character or a shadow will show itself as the part we are looking for.

For some patients, other techniques are more helpful in locating images of parts. For example, if you think about major events in your life, you may be able to visualize the scene of one or more of those events in detail. High school or college graduation, the birth of your child, your wedding, or achieving something for which you worked hard are good examples. In such scenes, you may be able to visualize yourself from outside yourself. Thus, you may visualize not only the triumphant moment but also an image of yourself as you experience that moment.

Other events that you might visualize in detail could be traumatic, such as the death of a loved one, a major argument, a military battle, a beating you received or witnessed when you were a child, and so on. In any of these memories, you might also be able to visualize yourself in the scene. If so, that is an example of a part or self-state of the sort with which Parts Psychology works. The parts therapist will guide you in having a conversation with such a part.

These are the parts of you that need to be healed—except for those with healthy, positive memories of the sort mentioned in an earlier paragraph. Therapy aims to help the patient discover the events that created a problem part. The next step is to neutralize the negative emotions and sensations still attached to the memories of those events. The result is that the part becomes centered rather than extreme. When that part and others become centered, so does the patient.

The Treatment Protocol

The standard treatment protocol for Parts Psychology can be simply stated, although it is often much more complex in application. The major elements are:

1. Define the problem (i.e., help the patient to describe the problem in specific rather than general terms).

2. Find the part that carries the problem (e.g., find the angry part, the depressed part, etc.).

3. Elicit the autobiographical memories that are the foundation for the problem.

4. Neutralize the problem memories through visualizing the part releasing the negative emotions and sensations.

The Parts Psychology protocol for standalone traumatic events such as childbirth varies somewhat from the standard protocol because we do not have to seek out the historical incidents that underlie the patient's emotional issues. We already know them. In Catherine's case, the issues were rejection by her mother and the 36 hours of labor. The focus of the therapy was narrowly defined as the set of negative emotions and sensations linked to the traumatic experiences. Consequently, we moved directly to the process of locating the parts in distress and healing them. We set the work within a narrative of significant events whose elements included establishing the normal context, telling the story of the trauma, and re-turning the story to a new normal context.

Unburdening and Neutralizing

The most important healing intervention in Parts Psychology is that of *unburdening*. It is a concept developed by Richard C. Schwartz in his *Internal Family Systems* therapy, although Helen Watkins's concept of *The Silent Abreaction* might be considered a precursor.[4] The basic idea is that, over time, internal parts develop burdens as the result of a patient's life experiences. Burdens could be things like depression, phobias, rage, or extreme beliefs. Healing a patient of these issues means unburdening the parts that carry the burdens.

Parts Psychology makes explicit that unburdening is achieved through *neutralizing* the memories that create the burden of pain or negative energy. (Elsewhere, I describe cases where positively experienced events also require neutralization.) A truly neutral memory can be likened to a high school history text in which reading the text produces no arousal of any sort; it is merely a black and white recording of factual information.

Unburdening a part of its rage might require neutralizing the memories of multiple beatings by a father. Unburdening depression might include neutralization of memories of multiple losses (e.g., deaths or other separations from significant people) during childhood and later. The part carries the burden on behalf of the person. The person benefits when the part releases its burden.

The therapy produces neutral memories out of painful ones through ritual or other symbolic visualizations of the burdened part releasing the attached negative emotions or sensations. Normally, the therapist will guide or assist the patient in the visualization. Sometimes, patients accomplish the neutralization of memories through visualizing something as simple as throwing the negative emotions in the trash. Most, however, seem to benefit from a more elaborate ritual. Here are three examples of such rituals. In each of these examples, the therapist narrates the intervention for the patient while the patient directs the part in the release of its negative energy.

(1) Visualize the part standing in a waterfall and notice how sometimes there are drops of water and sometimes mist and sometimes a powerful pouring of water. Let the water flow over, around and through her. Notice how the part's hair is plastered to her head and her clothes are stuck to her skin. Ask her to locate where it is within her that she stores the problem memory and then ask her to feel the water dissolving the pain and negative emotions connected to the memory. Notice how the negative emotions dissolve in the water and the water washes them out of her. You may even notice how the water around her is discolored as the dissolved negative emotions are washed away. As the water continues to wash away her anger [or fear, sadness, etc.] you may notice how it gradually becomes clear again as the memory is washed clean.

(2) Visualize a bonfire for the part and ask him to stand in front of it. Then ask him to locate where it is within him that he stores the painful memories. Now ask him to reach inside of himself and lift out the negative emotions [or negative energy] and throw them into the fire. As the fire touches them, you can see them burst into flame and be totally incinerated. Ask him to go back for more and keep repeating the action until all of the negative emotions and sensations that were attached to the memories are entirely consumed in the fire.

(3) Visualize the part standing in an open field and bring up a powerful wind to blow over,

around, and through her. Ask her to locate where it is within her that she stores the memory and ask her to feel the wind scouring the memories and washing them clean of fear and anger [or sadness, shame, etc.]. As the wind breaks up the fear and anger into tiny particles, you may notice that as the wind blows away from her it is darker because it is blowing away the particles of those emotions like dust or sand. Let the wind continue to blow until the memory is just a neutral memory with no particular emotion attached to it.

There is one additional intervention that was especially important in the work with Catherine. Here, I call it a *rescue*, but it is common to many different therapies and probably originates in work by hypnotherapists in the 19th century.5 It involves the patient visualizing the rescue of an internal part from a painful place to a safe place. In Catherine's therapy, the safe place was always the visualized scene of her son's nursery. She would recall a painful scene and then rescue the version of herself that she found in that scene by taking the part's hand and stepping from the traumatic scene to the calm scene of the nursery. The rescue contributes to neutralizing the painful memory although it is generally not enough by itself to accomplish the task.

Chapter 4
Session 2: Attachment Loss.

Our first session revealed that Catherine had experienced a serious attachment wound through her mother's response to the news of her pregnancy. Mother and daughter had been best friends all of Catherine's life. It was a tremendous blow to Catherine to find her mother rejecting her rather than sharing in her happiness. When she shared the news of her pregnancy with her parents, her father smiled and congratulated her with a hug. Her mother, however, was glum. She seemed to be irritated rather than joyful. She did not congratulate her; nor did she smile and hug her. All she said was "You timed that perfectly!"

Catherine didn't know what her mother meant, but assumed that she was irritated that Catherine hadn't consulted her on the timing of the planned pregnancy. After that meeting, her mother avoided Catherine. She did not call her and did not speak to her even at the gym where each of them did daily workouts. Throughout the pregnancy, Catherine's mother maintained her silence. The daily talks, lunches and shopping together ended abruptly. Catherine felt isolated and abandoned, and mourned the connection she once had with her mother. She felt alone and unsupported throughout her pregnancy.

Because I thought that this lost connection with her mother might have somehow contributed to Catherine's difficulties in childbirth and her later postpartum depression, we focused first on the trauma of her mother's abandonment before moving on to the physical trauma of the difficult birth. My goal at this point of the therapy was to begin to engage Catherine with those parts of herself that carried the various sources of pain: sadness, disappointment, attachment loss, anger, etc.

I wanted to guide Catherine in beginning to connect with her internal self-states that needed to heal. The external self (observing self)—the Catherine with whom I was directly engaged in the therapy room—has only a limited ability to heal. The internal self-states that I call parts are the containers of emotional pain and it is they who must give up their distress. Thus, the next step was to guide Catherine in discovering that she had such internal parts and then to help her in communicating with them.

I asked Catherine to tell the story again of how her mother responded to learning of her pregnancy. The repeated telling helps both therapist and patient to focus on the most relevant aspects of the story. Here is how she began her story:

"I was excited when I told her I was pregnant. I thought she would be happy for me. But there was no congratulation, no smile, just her comment about me choosing the time for the baby. That was the first hurtful thing. The worst thing was seeing her at the gym and her not looking at me and ignoring me like she didn't know me. The second worst thing was not having her at my baby shower. I feel numb now eight months after my baby came when I think about those gym meetings.

"We're still not talking. When the baby was four months old, my husband wanted to take me out on our first date since the baby. She and my dad were coming over later in the week to watch the baby.

When I asked my mother if she could [also] babysit for me so I could make a [doctor's] appointment, she said no. And she wanted to know every detail about why I needed help, like she had to judge whether I needed help or not. When we came home [from our date], the baby was crying and they were upset. My mother was flustered and my dad was trying to calm the baby. I said maybe it was because the baby wasn't used to them, since he hardly ever saw them. My mother just cursed and walked out. I haven't talked to her since."

Because Catherine was angry with her mother, I suggested that a good place to start parts therapy would be with her feeling of that anger. I asked her to think about her mother and check her emotions and body sensations. Immediately, she felt angry and located its strongest manifestation in her face. In order to begin the process of working with her internal parts, I asked her to speak, silently or aloud, to the sensation in her face and request that it make itself stronger. The result was that her face sensation increased and she felt her anger even more strongly. From a parts perspective, the important thing was that an internal self-state was responding to Catherine's request. Communication had begun.

Next, I guided Catherine in asking the sensation to "step back." The sensation lessened. Catherine asked the part to "step forward" again. The result was that the face sensation increased once more. We now had three requests of the unseen part and three positive responses. It was time to look for an internal image of the angry part so that we could work with it directly.

The purpose of requests to make a sensation stronger or to step back or step forward is to increase the separation of the part from the core self. For most people, talking to a part of themselves and coaching the part to respond is an unusual experience. Both the patient and the part go through a short learning process before they are able to communicate mind to mind. While it can be effective to speak directly to a sensation and to ask that it present itself as an image, I have found that more patients respond easily to the visualization request when these additional steps are added.

Surprisingly, when Catherine spoke to the face sensation and asked for an image of it, an image of her mother rather than an image of herself appeared. This sort of response, where the object of the anger appears rather than the angry part, is not unusual. When it happens we simply take another step or two to find the part we are looking for. What was unusual, however, was the appearance of the image of Catherine's mother. The image was that of a younger mother, perhaps in her 40s rather than her 60s, and her hair was wild and waving. When Catherine examined the wild movements of her mother's hair more closely, she discovered that the hair consisted of snakes, imitating the mythical Greek image of Medusa, a monster whose gaze turned mortals into stone. When asked, the image stated that her name was indeed *Medusa* and that she was Catherine's mother. Medusa was a *mother introject,* about which I will say more below.

In order to continue with Catherine's anger, we asked Medusa if she knew the angry part. She did. And she agreed to draw that part into Catherine's imagery. [Note: an ellipsis (...) below indicates where I have excluded my question before Catherine's response.] Catherine described this part as looking like her, but younger—aged 22 versus Catherine's 34. "But she has two sides, a blank slate—and that's my numbness—and the other side is red—that's my anger. She has long blonde hair like before my baby. ...Yes, she knows Medusa, my mother. She has known her forever. She feels fear toward her and also a love attachment and anger. ...Yes, she knows both Medusa and the outside mother. They are the same, yet different. Medusa is the awful one. I see my mother with three sides: her body with normal looks, Medusa as the awful one who is scary—she wears red clothing—and third is the kind mother, calm and wearing light-colored clothing."

We called the angry part *Catherine 22* to distinguish her from both the outside Catherine, who talked to me in my office, and other, inside, Catherines we might meet later. We wanted to reduce Catherine 22's anger so that Catherine would benefit through a reduction of *her* anger. We asked the angry part to share her most disturbing memory of her mother. The scene that came to Catherine's mind was that of being "very round" in late pregnancy, wearing workout clothes in the gym. Her mother was there, too, but she was ignoring Catherine. "She acted like she didn't know me."

This scene is one that repeated itself many times during the pregnancy because both mother and daughter went daily to the same gym. Still, I will speak of it as if it were a single event. I was surprised that this memory scene was the earliest held by the angry part. I expected something from Catherine's childhood because anger is a normal part of human experience throughout life. I expected that we would find previous autobiographical memories later in the therapy. However, because the focus of our work was the set of events surrounding Catherine's pregnancy and childbirth, we might safely choose to temporarily ignore anger-producing experiences from Catherine's younger ages.

Freestanding and Stuck-in-the-Memory Parts

The image of a pregnant Catherine in the gym is what I call a *stuck-in-the-memory part* because it is connected to a particular time and place in Catherine's history. I have sometimes called such parts *memory-scene parts*. Such parts often have no other memory than the one in which they are located. These scenes always represent high-energy moments in a patient's life.

In contrast, Catherine 22 is a *freestanding part* because she has been emancipated from enclosure in any particular memory scene. She presumably has a full range of autobiographical memories that begins in Catherine's childhood. Catherine 22 is a resource available to us again and again if we decide to explore earlier life events that might contribute to Catherine's current problems. The stuck-in-the-memory part in the gym is important because healing it is the first step in reducing Catherine's anger with her mother (and possibly her postpartum depression).

Catherine 22 reported distress at a 10 on the 0-10 SUD ("Subjective Units of Disturbance") scale that we used to measure parts' distress. Whatever the beginning level of emotional pain, the only acceptable level at the conclusion of work with a memory is a SUD level of zero, meaning that the part we healed would then feel neutral about the memory.

Catherine began healing the stuck-in-the-memory part by revealing to the part the ultimately positive outcome of having a healthy and thriving baby. By giving this information to the part, we aimed to reduce her negative energy and help her to be more flexible in working with us. The pregnant part in the gym was unaware of events later in time than the scene in the gym that held her. (Not all stuck-in-the-memory parts are so limited; sometimes they can have significant memories beyond the traumatic event in which they are located.)

Catherine chose a wind metaphor to neutralize the negative energy attached to the gym memory. She asked the pregnant part to focus on the location within her where she stored her "upset" for her mother's behavior and then to notice how the wind Catherine brought broke up the feelings into tiny particles and blew them out and away from her. Catherine visualized a powerful wind blowing over, around and through Catherine 22 and visualized as well how the particle-full wind was darker as it blew away from the part. After a single pass of the intervention, the SUD measure of Catherine 22's distress for this scene fell from 10 to 4. When asked, the part indicated that the SUD level hadn't reduced to zero because she still needed answers as to why her mother behaved in this way.

Across many contexts and situations, parts frequently express the desire to understand why a distressing event occurred, or why a hurtful person acted as she did. As humans we want to think there is some rational purpose behind painful events. In Parts Psychology, however, the therapist normally sidesteps these questions whenever possible in the interest of therapeutic efficiency. In fact, insight and understanding more often come *after* rather than before healing. For this reason, Catherine suggested to the part that the answers would eventually come, but for now she could help herself and Catherine best by first letting go of her distress. Catherine repeated the wind visualization twice more before the part rated it zero on the SUD scale.

Catherine completed the session's work with two other interventions. First, she quickly visualized for the pregnant part the step-by-step process of the baby's delivery and, second, she rescued the part from the gym scene and moved her, no longer pregnant, to Catherine's present-time nursery. (I do not know at what place in the intervention the image of the part changed from pregnant to not pregnant.)

My notes at the end of the session suggested the following for possible attention in the next session: rescue any other stuck-in-the-memory parts that might be stuck in the pain of the mother's silence; work to produce additional healing of Catherine 22's anger; unmask and remove the costume of the mother introject (described below); and begin processing Catherine's traumatic memories of giving birth. All of these thoughts were tentative, just possibilities for continued therapy, depending upon Catherine's state when I saw her at the beginning of the next session. Overall, I was pleased with our progress. Catherine was comfortable with this new way of relating to herself and not at all surprised to discover that parts of her could "talk" back to her.

Chapter 5
Session 3: Unmasking the Introject

Catherine began our third session by observing that "I've been looking at my baby now with more joy as my depression begins to lift. It's hard to explain. It's not that I wasn't joyful with him before but it's different now. I'm feeling energy now when I'm with him and I enjoy playing with him more. He makes me laugh and that feels good."

Because we had been successful in reducing the antipathy Catherine felt for her mother, it seemed reasonable to continue that process before beginning our work on the childbirth trauma. It seemed that Catherine's relationship with her mother was an important element in her continuing postpartum depression and possibly part of the foundation for the great distress and pain she felt giving birth to her son. For this reason, we returned to work with Medusa, the mother introject that had been a part of Catherine's inner world since childhood. First, however, a short detour to explain introjects.

Introjects

Introjects are constructions in a person's (usually a child's) inner world that represent some of the characteristics of a significant figure in her or his life. The problem introjects primarily differ from other internal parts in that they refuse or are unable to acknowledge that they are a part of the whole person; instead, they insist that they *are* the person after whom they are patterned. In my experience with this type of introject, most have a continuing negative impact on patients' lives for as long as they are unhealed. For example, they may increase anxiety, maintain unhealthy levels of self-blame, cause oversensitivity to criticism, and contribute to other problem emotions and beliefs.

The primary function of a problem introject seems to be that of maintaining a constant internal reminder that the person represented by the introject is someone to be wary of, someone whose power and control over the child is always relevant. Thus, the child learns to be wary of the parent's potential threat even in the absence of the parent. While not all introjects are parental introjects like Catherine's Medusa, I will describe them here as parental introjects for ease of discussion.

Powerful persons in a child's life such as parents seem most likely to be introjected when they are both unpredictable and threatening. Physical and emotional abusiveness are additional characteristics in a parent that could easily lead to the appearance of a negative introject in a child. When a parental introject is created, not all of the parent's characteristics are introjected, just those that require a continuing wariness.

An introject is then, like many other internal parts, a kind of stereotyped construction. In a few cases, a patient might introject positive characteristics of a parent and thereby create an internal self-state that is nurturing and helpful. That was not true of Catherine's Medusa. With a different patient of mine, an example of such a case is one where there was a positive father introject whose only function seemed to be to provide companionship to a toddler part. In that patient's outside life, the father had disappeared by the time the patient was three or four years old.

In another case, a patient had created a manager part—one that supervised and looked after the patient's set of internal child parts—based upon certain positive strengths of the mother. The image of this positive introject was that of the mother and it identified itself with the name of the mother. However, there is an important difference between this case and the problem introjects of the sort represented by Medusa. In the manager case, the positively motivated introject recognized that it was a part of the patient and not a separate entity. In the case of Medusa and similar negative introjects, the parts present themselves to the patient as if they were actually the parent. They resist the idea that they are part of the patient.

When eliciting memories from a Medusa sort of introject, the therapist will initially find its memories to be similar to the memories of more ordinary internal parts in that they appear to record significant events in the patient's life. But there is an important difference. The problem introject presents these "autobiographical" memories as if they were experienced by the parent, not the patient. For example, a patient eliciting memories from a six-year-old part might recall an incident where the mother was "mean," publicly scolding and spanking her in a department store. The mother's actions might bewilder the child—e.g., "What did I do wrong?" When the story of the same event is collected from the mother introject, the introject might emphasize how the child was "bad" for being noisy or for embarrassing the mother in the store.

Thus, the patient has unconsciously reconstructed the memories to present the mother's presumed point of view, including the emotions and motives that explain her actions. But these are just guesses. Because the introject's explanations are efforts by the child to make sense of the parent's actions and not the actual parent explaining herself, they might or might not accurately present the mother's point of view at the time. They can only be hypotheses (guesses).

In theory, the disturbing memories of a parental introject can be neutralized in the same way as those of other parts. In practice, however, the work is quite difficult and confusing. At the outset, attempts to neutralize the presumed memories of the introject are inconsistent with the healing protocol. Unburdening aims to heal a part of its burden of negative emotions. An introject like Medusa, however, presents itself as separate from the patient, presumably with its own burden—one that does not belong to the patient. Hence, the patient cannot unburden her mother's pain.

Of course, we know as therapists that the introject is not the actual mother. Unfortunately, it is some-times difficult to convince the patient of this. It is even more difficult to convince the internal self-states. They are actually the cause of the patient's difficulty. After many hours of frustrating work with introjects that could not be easily unburdened or convinced that they were not the person they presented themselves to be, I found that the simplest and most efficient way to work with introjects was to unmask them by asking them to remove their parent costumes. We could then heal the revealed child part that wore the mask and costume. In so doing, the therapist quickly dispenses with significant barriers to healing the patient in a timely manner.

Unmasking Medusa

Our initial interaction with Medusa was enough to make clear that this part viewed itself as Catherine's actual mother and thus different from other parts that made up Catherine's internal world. Her earliest memories were of Catherine behaving in an undisciplined way. She presented as threatening and fearful to other parts. Rather than do a lengthy interview with Medusa while collecting the introject's jaundiced view of Catherine's life, I chose to shortcut the process by proceeding directly to unmasking her and moving on to heal the likely child part who wore the Medusa costume.

Unmasking an introject by directing the hidden child part to remove its costume is a routine part of Parts Psychology. The following steps are usually sufficient to accomplish the task.

1. Thank the introject for being a part of the patient's life and for helping the patient to survive into adulthood.

2. Congratulate the introject for doing such a good job of protecting the patient.

3. Praise the introject for being an outstanding actor (in portraying the parental role).

4. Assert that the introject is a part of the patient and not separate from the patient.

5. Direct the child beneath the costume to unzip or otherwise remove its costume or mask

and just *be* the young patient inside the costume.

The first steps of thanking, congratulating, and praising the introject aim to create a positive relationship with the introject, one that fosters cooperation. Asserting that the introject is a part of the patient and not separate from the patient is intended to weaken the introject's belief that it is indeed the outside person it represents, in this case, Catherine's mother. And then, before there is further discussion about whether the introject is a part of the person or separate from the person's parts, we move quickly to request the unmasking of the introject. This simple protocol has been successful with nearly all of my uses of it.

In the following paragraph I provide an example of the kind of ritual I suggest for unmasking an introject. After each sentence I pause so that the patient can repeat (silently or aloud, depending upon the patient's preference) my words or ideas to her internal image of the introject.

Thank you for helping me to grow into adulthood. Because of you I have succeeded in surviving through difficult times. Congratulations! Without you, I could not have survived. You are absolutely the best at what you do. Congratulations also on being the very best actor ever. And you have played a very difficult and exhausting role. The role you played was that of being my mother and you convinced all the other parts that you are her. But you can retire now, because you have succeeded in your job. You have guided me into adulthood. You are wearing a mother costume but you are not my mother. You are me, a younger me. It's time now for you to take off your mask and costume and just be the younger me behind the mask and under the costume. So please just go ahead and unzip the costume and step out of it or pull it over your head, and let me see the *me* behind the mask.

The result of the intervention was that Medusa transformed herself into a little girl of about three years of age. Catherine visualized her as unzipping her costume and stepping out of it. It was a simple intervention, easily accomplished. Its purpose was to release Catherine from the internal oppression and consequent fear she had of Medusa's displeasure. A secondary purpose was to bring all of Catherine's parts together onto the same team, with the understanding that all of them were parts of the whole person.

The final step in healing an introject is to unburden whatever might oppress the newly revealed child part. When Catherine asked if she had any bad feelings or memories she wanted to heal, the three-year-old did not respond. She seemed to be fine. However, just to be safe, Catherine visualized blowing a gentle wind over, around and through the image of the little girl and coached her to let the wind carry away any "bad feelings" she might have. After this intervention, Catherine observed, "She feels safe now. She's carrying a stuffed monkey." Catherine went on to explain that she was an adult now and she would care for the little girl. If she wanted to do so, the little girl could look through Catherine's eyes at Catherine's new baby. The three-year-old, however, just wanted "to play." I have found that "wanting to go play" is the best indication that a child part has healed.

Reducing Catherine's Hurt and Anger

Once Medusa was unmasked, we could return to work with angry Catherine 22 and then move on to the childbirth trauma. Catherine easily located again the image of Catherine 22 and asked her to identify the most disturbing memory she had of her mother. It was that of her mother not being there for her pregnancy. Catherine 22 was very angry with the mother, with a SUD ("Subjective Units of Disturbance") level at the maximum of 10. Her anger was mixed with hurt—because "she had to do it all alone." Her hurt also reached a 10 on the SUD scale. Her mother did not support her, was not by her side, and did not share her knowledge of childbirth with her. In response to Catherine's request, Catherine 22 readily agreed to unburden her hurt and anger.

Catherine chose an ocean metaphor to neutralize memories, first visualizing Catherine 22 in the sea with the waves flowing gently over her to dissolve her hurt. After a few moments, Catherine reported that the hurt had reduced from a SUD of 10 to a 5 but Catherine 22 was blocked at 5 because of her anger. Next, Catherine asked the part to focus on her anger as she brought more ocean waves to wash away her negative emotions. That produced a SUD score of 2 for both hurt and anger.

Because it is usually helpful to encourage a part to say more about the feelings that prevent complete neutralization of particular memories, Catherine asked Catherine 22 to explain her remaining hurt and anger. The part responded that she was hurt because this was her only baby and she couldn't take back the experience; she would always be alone. Catherine explained that she would not be alone because they (self and part) would be together, and together they would remember what they shared.

With one more pass of the ocean intervention, the SUD level reached 1—which the part felt "in her eyes." Returning once more to the ocean, Catherine asked the part to open her eyes underwater and let the water dissolve the remaining negative emotion. Then, without an immediate check on the SUD level, she rescued the part to a safe place. She assured the part she would visit her there.

Before we could end the session, Catherine said that her throat felt "scratchy." When she checked inside to look for a possible source from among her internal parts, she found that the sensation originated with Catherine 22. To soothe her scratchy throat, Catherine visualized the part drinking hot tea and found that this was the intervention that finally reduced to zero the anger and hurt for her mother's absence.

This ended a session in which we focused almost exclusively on Catherine's issues with her mother. With a hurried ending to the meeting, I thought there might still be more work we needed to do with Catherine 22. If not, then I hoped we could now heal the specific traumatic moments Catherine revealed in the initial narrative. I also thought we might first have to find and unburden the part that continued to be fearful of the mother.

Chapter 6

Session 4: Neutralizing Traumatic Memories

At the beginning of the session I asked Catherine about the fear of her mother she had mentioned at the end of the last session. She said that while that is generally the feeling she had when thinking about her mother, she did not feel that today. Consequently, we could move directly to the planned work of neutralizing the traumatic memories identified in our first session. We would work with the stuck-in-the-memory parts from the narrative.

The first of these that readily came to mind was the part Catherine had either found or created when, not knowing "how to push," she visualized an image of herself pushing the baby through the birth canal. Her use of this intervention during delivery seems to have been spontaneous and illustrates how the creation of parts is a normal human process during times of need. Catherine easily found this stuck-in-the-memory part in her memory of the delivery room. Her pregnant self was working hard at pushing out her baby. She readily accepted Catherine's offer to neutralize the continuing pain she felt.

Catherine chose to place the image of herself in the shower and to use the imagery of flowing water as the healing intervention. The first pass of the visualization reduced the SUD level from 10 to 2. Catherine quickly followed that by sharing with the part the narrative of events from the intense labor scene through the successful delivery of her baby. She added a description of the experiences of going home from the hospital and taking care of her baby during the next eight months. This visualization, by providing the part with the rest of the story, reduced its SUD score to zero. Catherine then rescued the part from the scene altogether by visualizing taking her hand and stepping with her into Catherine's present-time nursery.

The next stuck-in-the-memory part Catherine chose to unburden was the image of herself on the following day. That was when she struggled with learning how to breastfeed her baby while feeling exhausted, lonely, inadequate and in significant pain—especially from her back. This time Catherine chose a fire metaphor to heal the painful memories. She visualized a bonfire for the part and imagined the stuck-in-the-memory Catherine reaching inside of herself, lifting out, and then throwing her distress from all sources into the fire for incineration. Within half a minute the pain had reduced from a SUD level of 8 or 9 to a level 1. The part indicated that it still had some distress because she felt "stuck" in her hospital bed; she couldn't move. When Catherine rescued her to the nursery-room safe place, the SUD reduced to zero

Seeking additional scenes to neutralize, I asked Catherine to think of the hospital again and share with me what she felt. She described a sensation in her throat that she interpreted as anxiety. When she asked for an image of that anxiety, what came to mind was an image of her attending nurse, looking down on her. She saw the nurse as viewed from her position in bed, looking up. The nurse was not anxious.

For situations like this, where the patient views an image of another person in a memory scene rather than an image of herself, there are a number of techniques available to locate the part. In this case, I suggested to Catherine that she speak to the nurse image and request of her that she speak to the Catherine in bed and ask this anxious part to step away from the body so that both Catherine and the nurse could see her. The nurse image did as requested, with the result that Catherine could now see an image of the anxious part of herself as well as the nurse. The nurse image was of no further value in the discussion.

Catherine could now describe the appearance of the anxious stuck-in-the-memory part we were looking for. She said, "I see myself in a hospital gown, with a puffy face, my hair still long and in a ponytail. She is the same age as me and she is exhausted and just drained more than anxious." Rather than use one of the standard wind, water, or fire metaphors to neutralize the memory of anxiety and exhaustion, Catherine chose to wrap up her negative emotions and knock them over the horizon with a baseball bat. In doing so, she demonstrated that unburdening parts through neutralizing memories does not always require complex visualizations. The puffy-eyed stuck-in-the-memory part now rated her SUD level at zero. As a final step, Catherine moved this part to the safe place of her current-time nursery. When I directed Catherine to think again of the hospital, she felt no other anxiety.

We returned then to the original narrative of the childbirth story so that Catherine could check for other still-disturbing memories. She quickly focused upon the stuck-in-the-memory image of herself in the birth tub at the moment of her greatest pain. It was also the moment of her greatest fear.

By now we had found a rhythm in our work: find the part, choose an unburdening ritual, and then neutralize the memory through carrying out the ritual. Catherine chose to return to wind imagery and visualized the stuck-in-the-memory part letting her fear and pain go to the wind that Catherine blew over, around, and through her. Within a few moments, Catherine checked with the part in the birth tub and found that her SUD level for the experience was down to 1. The part could not explain why it was not at zero. I coached Catherine to provide a strong blast of wind to this stuck-in-the-memory part to release the last of the negative energy and then to rescue the part to Catherine's favorite safe place, her nursery. Catherine followed my coaching, but then added, "She's in the nursery but she's drawn back to the memory scene—it's the water tub."

In this instance, my own anxiety about the approaching end of the session had caused me to rush Catherine before she had discerned what was causing the temporary block in the process. Catherine then added, "It's because she knows if she leaves the tub, it's the epidural [i.e., she would be given an epidural injection to ease the pain] and she doesn't want that." The solution was for Catherine to share with the part from the water tub a visualization of the entire set of experiences through the birth of the child and then to rescue her to the nursery. "She's okay now," said Catherine. The SUD value was zero. When Catherine checked her hospital memories again for any remaining anxiety or other problem moments, she could find none. It appeared that our work might be done.

At our next session, which I thought might be our last, I wanted to check the narrative once more for other disturbing memories.

other disturbing memories. I also wanted to check to see if her postpartum depression had lifted, and if not, to do whatever was needed to bring that about. Finally, I wanted Catherine to fill out another depression questionnaire so that we could check it against the one she filled out prior to our first session.

Chapter 7
Session 5: Examining Results

We began our fifth session with Catherine saying, "Telling the story is easier now. I talk to my friends about it without getting upset. One friend told me about her daughter giving birth in just 20 minutes. She helped deliver her daughter's baby in the bathroom before the ambulance arrived. Previously, I would have beaten myself up again after hearing her story, thinking 'just another case of popping it out.' I would have obsessed again over my difficulties. But I could be happy now for her. I just let go of my own pain. I don't feel upset or frustrated."

She talked some about her relationship with her husband, saying that interaction with him had been "a little bit stressful" during the week. "He doesn't hear me. He discounts it [i.e., Catherine's problems]. 'Just get over it; move on!'"

This reaction by her husband is a fairly common response by those who are frustrated by being unable to help their loved ones. So they urge them to act like nothing happened or to quit thinking about it. They may have handled their own issues by similarly suppressing them and may thus believe that others should also be able to do so. They really cannot understand until they are themselves overtaken by a trauma or a depression that seemingly has its own driving force. In fact, it is possible to eventually move on without healing the painful issues, but the life we move on to will likely be a life much less fulfilling than a life that has taken the time to heal.

On an upbeat note, Catherine noticed that she was now much less frustrated with her husband than she used to be. For example, she observed that he was a driven man, totally focused on his work, but a procrastinator at home. She had been asking him to fix, or have fixed, a garage door that would not open, requiring her to park in the driveway. "Four weeks ago I would have been yelling at him, really upset, thinking things can only get worse. Now I am much more calm. He's made the phone call and someone will fix it when they can."

In order to assess how complete the therapy might be, I asked Catherine to review the birth narrative. Her general comments were that "I don't feel the kind of pain I felt before. Then, I went straight to the pain—incredible pain! Now I see it—I view it like a movie—and I don't feel the pain." More particularly, I asked about the moment in the water tub. "At about 15 or 17 hours [of labor] I got into the birth tub. I thought it would be more comfortable. But it got worse. The pain and pressure in my back immobilized the lower half of my body. The pain pulled me toward a fetal position. I had a rag in my mouth for screaming. I thought it was going to be easier." The SUD measure for this most painful part of the narrative was now zero.

Catherine continued, "I kept asking every hour, 'How much longer?' I was stuck at five centimeters [birth would be at nine or 10 centimeters]. I got out [of the tub] at 18 hours [of labor], got an epidural. They changed the brand of epidural to find an effect. It didn't help. The anesthesiologist came every two hours. The doctor and the nurses were often down there checking, moving things around. I felt invaded—like an alien abduction—while being examined."

In retelling this part of the story Catherine seemed to be again feeling some distress. It was different from the pain she previously felt for her memories, but still disturbing. It was the sense of "being invaded." The examinations "down there" were the focus of her attention. The memory scene that came to mind was: "Me on the bed in stirrups. And stirrups for my hands too. You use them to pull yourself up and curled over, with the doctor down there." I suggested that Catherine say hello to this stuck-in-the-memory part and she did so. "She said she knows me, 'Catherine,' and she is also Catherine." When Catherine asked this part if she wanted help in getting out of this stuck place, the part replied, according to Catherine, "Yes, but I'm scared!" We did not collect an initial SUD rating for the scene, but a single pass of the wind intervention reduced the SUD to a 2 for her pain. A second pass reduced it to a SUD of 1.

Rather than continue with this reluctant release of pain, we turned to the matter of Catherine's feeling of a "sense of invasion." The stuck-in-the-memory part rated it at a level 8. Catherine used another wind intervention to neutralize this part's sense of invasion "wherever she felt it in mind or body." The result was a reduction of the SUD score to just "point five." When Catherine asked what else still bothered the part, she found that the part "wished she had been better able to help herself." She evidently felt some degree of helplessness.

This reply led me to ask Catherine to check with the stuck-in-the-memory part to see if she had any awareness of any internal force or pressure that might have caused difficulty in giving birth. I was interested to know if she had any awareness of Medusa, the mother introject we had worked with previously. But her answer was that she was calm in the labor room. "She has her husband there and her doula [labor coach] there but she still feels alone. She wishes her parents were there. Her dad texted her and her husband but there was nothing from her mother. She thinks she could have had an easier birth if her mother had just been in the waiting room or calling her."

[Jay]: "Ask her if she knows Medusa."
[Catherine]: "No, she doesn't know Medusa."
[Jay]: "Ask her if she had any sense that she was being punished."
[Catherine]: "Yes, she feels like she was being punished; she said so, but she doesn't know why, when she had done so much to do it right."
[Jay]: "Please ask her if she can think of any reason for which she might be punished."
[Catherine]: "No, she doesn't know why. She doesn't think she did anything wrong."
[Jay]: "What about her mother?"
[Catherine]: "Yes, she thinks that her *mother* thinks she did something wrong."

Catherine chose another wind intervention to neutralize the feelings of being alone, abandoned, and helpless. Within a few moments the SUD level reduced to 1. Next, hoping that a rescue would dispose of the remaining SUD energy, Catherine rescued the stuck-in-the-memory part to her current-time nursery. She found all the other parts there, too—those Catherine had previously moved to this safe place— five or six of them. They were taking turns holding the baby. [Notice that this is an internal fantasy. Catherine is talking about the activities among rescued parts in their fantasy nursery.]

Catherine continued, "She was able to see that I was there holding the baby and the other parts were there, too, and she was able to know how it all happened, so I didn't have to visualize the birth process for her." Like the other parts rescued to the nursery, this part was no longer pregnant. For the newly arrived part, the SUD score for pain was zero. The same was true for the sense of being invaded. Finally, she no longer felt lonely, abandoned, or helpless. She felt "no distress of any kind."

Before Catherine left the office, I asked her to take the same depression screen she had filled out before our first session. This is the CES-D, a public domain document. She now scored a six in comparison to the 22 she scored before therapy began. She was now well below the depression cutoff score of 15. We would check this depression screen again at our final session. We would also look for any residual of Catherine's traumatic feelings that we might have so far missed. Finally, we would check on Catherine's anger toward her mother because their relationship had been a major component in both Catherine's anger and her depression.

Chapter 8
Session 6: Review and Consolidate

As we began our sixth and final session, Catherine smiled comfortably and said "I feel good! I feel good!" We met this time for 90 minutes rather than the standard fifty because there were so many things to review. I asked about how she was doing in her relationship with her mother. She still had not seen her in several months. She went on to say:

> For so long I felt dependent upon approval from my mom. There was always lots of criticism from both of my parents for the career plans I made. For example, my mom would say, "Oh, that's too hard. You'll spend all your time working. When I finally chose my major in college and did what I thought best for me, she said nothing. She didn't attend my first graduation from college and it was an ordeal to get her to come to my next [MBA] graduation. She's never really been there for things that were really important to me. I'm just now connecting the dots. Until just now I didn't realize that her not being there for my birth isn't anything new. I still haven't seen her. There is still a teeny, teeny part of me that thinks [giving birth] would have been easier if she had been there. My dad comes by to see the baby every week. He thinks I don't need help, that I don't need support, that I can do anything I want.

Listening to Catherine, I could readily hear that she had made new insights, had "connected the dots" in a new way, and benefited from a new perspective in thinking about her mother. But she still wasn't fully okay with her current situation with her mother. That became obvious when she said, "Look at my hands! They are sweating! Just talking about Mom makes my body feel heated."

This sweaty-palms relationship with thoughts about her mother, however, was not the result of her mother's actions related to her giving birth. It was a long-held relationship surviving from the past. This became clear as we reviewed the major points we had covered in her narrative and in the therapy. As I listed those points, Catherine responded with a description of her current feelings. The first point was her mother's response of being angry rather than happy about Catherine's pregnancy. Catherine now felt "nothing;" it "was just something that happened." That is, she was neutral for the experience—the goal of the neutralization rituals. The relevant internal parts had been unburdened.

Over lunch with her mother when Catherine was two to three months pregnant, her mother had been "mean" and "bossy." Catherine had tried to tell her mother to be easier on her so that she could have a stress-free pregnancy. Her mother had responded by angrily insisting that she would say whatever she wanted to say. Catherine observed, "I'm not angry but there's a thing in my throat—like my throat starts to close in. There are more things I could have said, but didn't. I could have said, 'Look, you can't talk to me this way; I'm pregnant! I need to be stress-free for my baby!' I could have said more. The back of my throat closes in when I think of how I should have spoken more sternly, been more demanding of my need that she not be mean to me."

After that lunch, mother and daughter did not speak again except on one other occasion, when, together with her husband, she met for lunch with her mother and father. She had tried to mend things, but she was also trying to decide whether to invite her mother to her baby shower. The lunch was miserable and her mother was "negative and critical" about anything Catherine had to say. She decided not to invite her mother, knowing how easily her mother's negative attitude "could have ruined the baby shower for everyone." But now she was no longer upset about either this lunch or the silence that lasted until her baby was born.

Regarding the sudden ending of all communication with her mother, where previously they had talked up to several times daily and exchanged a steady flow of texts, Catherine said, "I don't feel angry or sad. I wish it were otherwise but it doesn't bother me." In sum, most of the problems with her mother leading up to the birth of the baby seem to have been neutralized. The remaining issues with her mother appear to be holdovers from previously unrecognized issues that had characterized the mother-daughter relationship for most or all of Catherine's life.

Returning to the narrative, the birth tub pain was no longer disturbing. Nor was the emotionally difficult and guilt-producing decision to ask for an epidural. Her mother had emphasized that only "weak women" chose to take an epidural. Strong women did childbirth naturally! Although the epidural didn't actually help much, asking for it caused Catherine to initially feel guilt and a sense of failure. Freeing herself from her mother's judgments seems to have freed her also from her guilt for not following her mother's guidelines for successful childbirth. We did not work directly on this guilt. Probably, the work we did to transform Medusa, the critical mother introject, helped Catherine to be free of the guilt. In fact, I believe that the unmasking of the introject was the single most significant thing we did to relieve Catherine of her distress over her mother's actions and inactions during the pregnancy.

In a similar way, choosing to ask for a C-section (which she did not actually get) led Catherine to experience guilt and a sense of failure. Now, "I feel fine knowing that I asked. At the time I thought I was going to die. I knew the baby was safe because I could hear his heartbeat. When I asked for it, that's when they told me to wait, that 'We can see hair.' My doula [birth coach], the nurses, the doctor all had confidence in me. But I had none. I decided to keep trying. The water broke at the end of the 35th hour and that's when things speeded up."

Regarding her memory of pushing out the baby by visualizing herself doing so, "I kinda think, 'I did it! I pushed the baby out! I made it through all those hours!' [Tears.] These are tears of relief. And pride. *I* was able to bring the baby to birth! *I* was able to have a healthy and happy baby!" Catherine had transformed her traumatic event from failure into triumph.

Other painful memories were also transformed. What was once an "alien invasion" of her body "down there" was now "just a medical procedure." Similarly, the memories of her first day after the birth, when she continued to be in significant physical pain and stressed with the difficulties of breastfeeding, were now quite differently viewed. "I don't feel sad. Now that I look at it now, I feel happy I have a baby I was able to breastfeed in the hospital and lucky I could stay four days [due to the baby's jaundice] and get extra care from the nurses to help me with breast-feeding before I took him home."

Catherine spoke now of the absence of her mother when she gave birth as factual rather than painful: "She wasn't there and that's just the way it was." Her next words made it clear that she now focused upon what she *had* rather than what she *didn't* have: "My husband was so supportive. He was there the whole time. He was even delusional because he didn't eat in all that time." Still, she wasn't quite neutral for her mother's absence, although she saw herself in a new and positive light:

It sucks that she wasn't there. But I look at it now that I did this huge thing without her. If I can do *that,* I can do *anything!* [Tears.] My tears go back to what so many people have told me: 'Thirty-six hours! If you can do *that,* you can do *anything!*' All my life I did everything with her. I found I don't need her for every-thing like I always did. I have had a hard time giving myself credit for anything and now I've done a huge thing! By myself! Now I want to embrace the thirty-six hours like a battle wound, a scar I can show off to someone. Gosh, I did this!

I asked Catherine whether perhaps her mother did her a favor by not being there. Her response was, "I hear your question now with a realization—right at this moment—that in a way she did. If you asked me that before the [therapy], I would have said, 'It hurts my soul!'"

I was curious about the status of the many stuck-in-the-memory parts that Catherine had rescued to her safe place: the baby's nursery at a time shortly after she brought her son home. She had just shared with me that she kept "in my mind the imagery of all the little parts in the nursery." I asked her to "go inside" and check on them to see if they were still there. In other cases, I have found that newly created stuck-in-the-memory parts often merge into a single entity. Catherine indicated that they were all still there. "I feel there are six of them. They are all sitting around in a circle watching the main part holding the baby. It feels like she's the stronger one of them all. I see her as the one that actually delivered the baby. Yes, she's the one I visualized pushing out the baby in the delivery room."

Appendix
PTSD and Postpartum Depression

At the conclusion of therapy, Catherine no longer met the criteria for either PTSD or postpartum depression. During the height of her pain, and ready for a C-section, she thought she was going to die. At that time, she felt intense fear and helplessness. After the therapy, however, she no longer had distressing memories of the events. She no longer avoided thoughts or conversations about her trauma and she was no longer numb and disinterested in the things she usually liked to do. She no longer tried to numb herself to the emotions previously aroused by her 36 hours of labor. She no longer experienced outbursts of anger and she now had no difficulty concentrating. Previously, Catherine had all of these symptoms and more. Her PTSD was gone.

Prior to the therapy, Catherine filled out the depression screen I ask all my patients to complete. Her gross score placed her in the moderate range of clinical depression. The questionnaire is a screen rather than a diagnostic instrument and its findings must be backed up by clinical observation to substantiate a diagnosis. My interest, however, was always in helping Catherine to process her traumatic labor and delivery, rather than achieving a precise diagnosis. Consequently, I did not directly address her depression symptoms in therapy. I expected them to diminish as the result of the therapy and they did so.

The instrument is the Center for Epidemiologic Studies Depression Scale (CES-D). It is a public domain document and can be freely downloaded from the internet. Catherine's initial score was 22, an indication of moderate depression. The cut-off score for mild depression is 15. Severe depression scores begin at 26. At the end of our fifth session, Catherine's score was six and at the end of our sixth and final session her score was four. I have included the full questionnaire below. Here, I will report on just four of the questions:

#4. I felt that I was just as good as other people.

#8. I felt hopeful about the future.

#12. I was happy.

#16. I enjoyed life.

These are the four "positive" items that are scored from zero to three, with a zero for "most or all of the time;" one for a "moderate amount of the time;" two for "a little of the time;" and three for "rarely or none of the time." The perfect score on these questions is zero.

Prior to our first session, Catherine scored herself as experiencing items 4 and 8 just "a little of the time" and rarely experienced the feelings in items 12 and 16 at all. She rated a total of 10 points on these four questions alone. After our last session, Catherine scored just three points total on these questions and four on the whole test.

She now indicated that she was happy "all or most of the time," and rated each of the other three statements "a moderate amount of the time." She explained why she didn't give herself a perfect score. "I felt I was just as good as other people" had never been "all or most" of the time. She strived to excel in school and career to overcome this sense of not being as good as others. Similarly, she had never been able to give herself full credit for her achievements and, as a consequence, wasn't sure if she could do so in the future. Thus, she wasn't entirely convinced that things would completely change. Finally, she said she was close to "all the time" for "I enjoyed life," but couldn't yet definitely say so. "But I am getting there. I will become happier." In sum, her postpartum depression was gone. The remaining issues were those which, although she made significant changes in them, were occasional issues she had had all of her adult life. They were not problematic enough that Catherine wanted to invest in additional sessions. She was pleased with what she had achieved.

Center for Epidemiologic Studies Depression (CES-D) Scale

Catherine's Initial Screen (Score=22)

1. I was bothered by things that usually don't bother me [One point].

2. I did not feel like eating; my appetite was poor [Zero].

3. I felt like I could not shake off the blues even with help from my family [Two points].

4. I felt I was just as good as other people [Two points].

5. I had trouble keeping my mind on what I was doing [One point].

6. I felt depressed [Two points].

7. I felt that everything I did was an effort [Two points].

8. I felt hopeful about the future [Two points].

9. I thought that my life had been a failure [Zero].

10. I felt fearful [Zero].

11. My sleep was restless [Zero].

12. I was happy [Three points].

13. I talked less than usual [Zero].

14. I felt lonely [Two points].

15. People were unfriendly [Zero].

16. I enjoyed life [Three points].

17. I had crying spells [Zero].

18. I felt sad [One point].

19. I felt that people disliked me [Zero].

20. I could not get "going" [One point].

Endnotes to Part 1

1 Noricks, Jay (2011). *Parts Psychology: A trauma-based, self-state therapy for emotional healing.* Los Angeles & Las Vegas: New University Press LLC.

2 See Watkins, J.G. & Watkins, H.H. (1997). *Ego states: Theory and therapy.* New York: WW Norton; Schwartz, R.C. (1995). *Internal Family Systems therapy.* New York: Guilford Press; Stone, H. & Winkelman, S. (1989). *Embracing ourselves: The voice dialogue manual.* Mill Valley, CA: Nataraj Publishing; Assagioli, R. (1965). *Psychosynthesis: A manual of principles and techniques.* New York: Penguin Books; Rowan, John (1990). *Subpersonalities: The people inside us.* London & New York: Routledge.

3 Prince, M. (1925). The problem of personality: How many selves have we? *Pedagogical Seminary and Journal of Genetic Psychology, 32,* 266-292.

4 Watkins, H.H. (1980). The silent abreaction. *International journal of clinical and experimental hypnosis,* XXVIII, 101-113.

5 See, for example, the work of Pierre Janet, as described in: Henri Ellenberger (1970). *The discovery of the unconscious: The history and evolution of dynamic psychiatry.* New York: Basic Books.

Part 2

Excerpt of *Chapter One* from:

Parts Psychology: A Trauma-Based, Self-State Therapy for Emotional Healing

By

Jay Noricks PhD

New University Press LLC

www.newuniversitypress.com

Los Angeles • Las Vegas

Preface

There are 15 chapters in this book. Thirteen of them form its core. These 13 chapters describe the in-depth success stories of 12 previously troubled psychotherapy patients. The stories represent a blend between psychological case reports and anthropological, cultural narratives. Narrative description is the focus of the book. Theory is minimal except in the first and last chapters.

Taking the time to describe the inner worlds of troubled patients is consistent with an anthropological approach to understanding whole cultures. It is consistent with the way, as an anthropologist, I approached writing up the results of my fieldwork on a tiny island in Polynesia. My first publications aimed at describing and understanding the way my consultants understood their world: a Polynesian-English dictionary, a paper on the local meaning of "crazy," and a description of a method for eliciting native speaker models of thinking.[1] Only later did I write more theoretical papers.[2] Now, having changed careers from anthropology to psychotherapy, I follow a similar path of emphasizing description before theory. The book contains both but the theory is dependent upon the description.

In putting together these narratives, I aimed for two different but overlapping audiences. The first is the general reader with an interest in psychology, especially those with interests in the organization of mind and the process of psychotherapy. My hope is that readers will find the inner worlds described here, and the therapeutic changes made through work with these worlds, just as fascinating as I found them. The idea that we all have multiple personalities—but not a disorder of personalities—may at first be shocking. But the evidence for this normal multiplicity among relatively ordinary people is so powerful that even the most skeptical of readers may change their minds before finishing the book. Many readers may discover some of their own parts as they read the stories in the core chapters.

The second audience is the experienced, professional psychotherapist or counselor. Therapists are always looking for new and better ways to help their patients. This book provides a complete description of how to do therapy in a new way. My hope for professionals is that that they will find something here that they can use in their own work. First in *Chapter 1,* which provides an overview of the model, and then through commentary embedded in the narratives of *Chapters 2* through *14,* I try to make clear in step-by-step fashion how Parts Psychology works. A careful reading of the introduction, the commentaries on the narratives, and the concluding chapter should answer most technical questions professionals might pose if they decide to add parts therapy to their treatment frameworks.

Chapter 1

The Parts Psychology Treatment Model

Parts Psychology is both a way of doing psycho-therapy and a way of understanding the mind. It approaches the therapy of troubled individuals by suggesting that the normal personality is not unitary; instead, the normal sense we have of being a unitary *I* or *me* is an illusion. It seems to be a necessary illusion, but still an illusion. The actuality is that the self is an agglomeration of many selves, and whichever self speaks as the I on any given occasion may be different from the self or group of selves that speaks as the I on another occasion.

We recognize our natural multiplicity in the ordinary language we use to express ourselves. A frustrated employee might say, "A part of me wants to tell my boss to go to hell, but the rational part of me says I need this job." Someone with marital issues might say, "A part of me wants to leave, but another part is afraid to be alone." A friend with an addiction might say, "I can go for a few days without using, but then a part of me takes over and I find myself getting high all over again."

These parts are the focus of Parts Psychology. Calling them *parts* is consistent with our everyday language, but the professional literature provides many other terms as well, including *subpersonalities, sides, subselves, internal self-states, voices* and *ego states*. When these parts are extreme and capable of taking full control of the person, as in the case of dissociative identity disorder (formerly called multiple personality disorder), they are called *alters* or *alter personalities*. This book does not describe any cases of dissociative identity disorder. Each of the extended case descriptions that make up the body of the book is a study of the inner world of a person with normal personality structure.

The idea that the normal personality consists of parts is not a new one. Morton Prince, a 19th and early 20th century pioneer in the study of dissociative identity disorder, also explored the natural divisions of the normal personality. He called these normal parts *sides*. He made the point that the sides of normal personalities are not very different from the alters of dissociative identity disorder.[3]

We now know that the difference is that alter personalities can completely take control of a person and the person retains no memory for the episode once the alter personality has relinquished control.[4] However, with normal persons, parts blend with the self without taking complete control and the person remembers the behavior influenced by the part. Generally, a person is unaware of a part's blending, and whether the person is feeling anger, sadness, joy or some other emotion, the blending is so seamless that the person owns the experience entirely. She would say, for example, "I am angry," without any sense that the anger originated in a blended subpersonality.

Following the early appearance of ideas about the natural multiplicity of the self,[5] there was a long period of neglect as Sigmund Freud's psychoanalytic framework overwhelmed psychology's treatment programs. Modern psychology is only now beginning to focus on what some scholars understood a century ago about the organization of the mind.

Parts Psychology recognizes the importance of the previous generation of scholars but takes the knowledge of our divided minds a step further. What is new, and even startling for some, is that we can help people artificially separate their parts from the self in the therapy room and actually engage in conversations with these parts. In this way, because we are working directly with the parts of the self that are most problematic, therapy becomes much more efficient. Healing moves at a much faster pace.

Two other models of psychotherapy heavily influence Parts Psychology as presented in this book. The first is the Ego State therapy of John and Helen Watkins.[6] The second is Richard C. Schwartz's Internal Family Systems therapy.[7] These two approaches are similar in that subpersonalities are accepted as important and natural elements of the mind and are not interpreted in terms of the older, grand theories of psychodynamic writers.[8] Both accept subpersonalities as "part persons" with a sense of self, a sense of purpose, and a way of perceiving the world that is unique to each part. Both approaches work with the individual parts that carry the problems in order to alleviate the distress of the whole person.

The differences are minor. The Watkinses worked almost exclusively through hypnosis while Schwartz emphasizes work with the fully conscious person. Another difference is that Schwartz encourages the therapist to work through the observing self, coaching its interaction with subpersonalities. The Watkinses, on the other hand, emphasize direct interaction between therapist and parts while the patient is in a state of hypnotic trance. As an apparent consequence of bypassing the fully aware (i.e., non-hypnotized) person in working with parts, the Watkinses do not directly acknowledge the presence of a self that is different from parts.

Most of the interventions I emphasize in Parts Psychology are also found in the work of either or both of the above models, but there are some important differences. I have borrowed the most important of these interventions from the work of Richard C. Schwartz. This is the concept of *unburdening.*[9] It involves the use of symbolic visualizations to release the problem emotions and beliefs the patient brings to therapy.

I have added to the unburdening intervention the use of a measuring tool to determine the degree to which a part has completely unburdened itself. And I have made clear that unburdening is achieved through *neutralizing* the energy (emotions and sensations) attached to particular autobiographical memories. Finally, I have extended the concept of unburdening beyond work with negative emotions to include work with positive emotions or sensations, such as love and sexual arousal that can sometimes be problems for patients.

Like Schwartz, I find that formal hypnosis is unnecessary in work with patients' internal worlds. I did not use formal hypnosis with any of the case descriptions presented in this book, although when patients concentrate on their internal parts their experience is sometimes trancelike.

One major difference from other approaches is that I emphasize that parts appear in our lives naturally, as the result of a universal, developmental process. When we need to adjust to something new in our lives, whether it is something in our own development, such as puberty, or something in our external environment, such as the way we are parented, additional subpersonalities spontaneously appear, enabling us to adjust to our changed situations. Thus, as we grow and develop, new parts appear whenever our existing parts cannot easily deal with a new challenge. Parts Psychology holds that subpersonalities are the natural building blocks of the mind, and without their development, we would lack the essential human flexibility that has allowed us to adjust to virtually every social and physical environment our planet has to offer.

A second difference lies in my emphasis upon painful life experiences as the basis for the development of most subpersonalities and for the later negative consequences that bring our patients to therapy. This emphasis means that healing has to do with neutralizing the negative energy (e.g., anger, anxiety) that is attached to the remembered experiences. The result of this neutralizing is that the experiences will no longer negatively impact our patients' lives.

Internal parts develop in response to our need to adjust to our life circumstances and, once created, these parts specialize in containing the memories that have some similarity to the original experiences that brought the parts into being.

When the way our parts influence us becomes less helpful and more damaging to the way we function, it is essential to help them become more centered and flexible in their roles. Flexibility follows from neutralizing some or all of the emotional content of a part's set of memories, beginning with the earliest memories recorded in the memory set. The original painful events, sometimes so painful they should be called traumas, are the most important concerns of therapy. Until the memories of the original events are neutralized, many later painful events cannot be fully processed.

There are a few exceptions to the rule that subpersonalities appear in our lives in response to painful life experiences. Parts can also appear as the result of our experience of positive but novel life events. For example, one of my female patients developed a new part at the age of 10 when she met a boy who became a friend and introduced her to his world of video and computer games. This fun-loving part became an important aspect of her life, expanding its original function of adjusting to her new friend to many other situations where a joyful and energetic approach to life was appropriate.

With such positively functioning subpersonalities, there is no need for therapeutic intervention. In another case, discussed later in *Chapter 4*, the patient developed a part who found joy in helping others. In childhood, this was an endearing trait. In adulthood, however, this trait worked against her in the workplace, where the time she spent helping coworkers meant she was not finishing her own assigned tasks, ultimately leading to her being fired. In this case, change was necessary. The positive energy attached to the helper part's early experiences had to be neutralized before the part could become flexible enough to know when to give priority to the patient's own needs over the needs of others.

Case Example

In the following example, I sketch the inner world of a normal person with a small number of subpersonalities. My purpose is to give the reader a sense of how internal parts can be organized in a normally functioning person. I address many other questions raised by the case example in later chapters of the book. In this case, all of the patient's parts have names, although they evidently did not have names before we did the work to differentiate them from the self. I later learned that, on their own, the parts chose names as we sought them out and interviewed them.

Madeline, the patient, is a successful, 40-year-old professional woman with no outstanding psychological issues. She is a normal high-functioning person. She is the district sales manager for a multinational corporation. Madeline did not come to me for therapy for specific issues; instead, she wanted to get a better understanding of who she was. She said that she had read about the idea that everyone had internal subpersonalities, and if that were true, she wanted to know about hers. Except for helping Madeline differentiate her parts, I did no other therapeutic interventions with her. All she wanted to accomplish was to become acquainted with her internal world. We did the work without formal hypnosis. Simple absorption techniques were all that was necessary. An example of such a technique is, "Focus upon that feeling and ask it to give you a picture of itself." I describe additional techniques later in this chapter.

Madeline has just five internal parts, an unusually small number. Possibly, the small number is due to the relative absence of significant trauma in

Madeline's early life. There is a child, an adolescent, and three adults. The child is *Bunny* who presents herself as a six-year-old girl. Madeline believes that Bunny's internal image probably represents what she herself looked like as a child. Bunny is playful, relates well to Madeline's children, and loves animals. She often gives Madeline dreams because, she says, she does not have the vocabulary to communicate like a grownup. She claims to have the ability to retrieve all of Madeline's memories, including everything Madeline has ever read.

Bunny was the second of Madeline's internal parts to develop, appearing at the age of four when Madeline felt shut out from her grieving parents when her younger brother died. Incidentally, Bunny does not view Madeline's mother as her own mother, although she sees Madeline's father as her father. The closest Bunny has to a mother is *Vivian,* the system's internal manager. The two of them relate to each other, Madeline says, like a mother and daughter.

The adolescent is *Suzanne.* She presents herself as 14 years old. She developed during Madeline's tumultuous teenage years slightly before Vivian became active and began evolving toward her eventual role as the system manager. However, unlike Vivian, Suzanne did not rebel against the mother. Instead, she passively endured. She wanted to be pretty and desirable, while her mother regularly told her she was ugly and undesirable. The internal image Madeline has of Suzanne is that of a beautiful teenager with only a slight resemblance to Madeline. Suzanne is a romantic, given to reading romance novels. Among her functions are overseeing Madeline's appropriate dress and social etiquette. Suzanne is quite vain.

The three adults are Vivian, aged 44, the internal manager; *Janice,* aged 33, the worker and taskmaster; and *Sally,* aged 34, the worrier. Janice and Sally's ages are approximate; they do not claim an exact age. Vivian ages along with Madeline. Vivian says she first appeared in Madeline's life at about 10 years of age but did not become active until slightly after Suzanne, the adolescent, appeared, perhaps at 14 or 15. Vivian developed in response to the need to stand up to a dominating mother.

The teenage years were difficult, full of the mother's verbal, and occasionally physical, abuse. It was the time when Vivian was most angry, and led to her becoming the system's anger manager. The mother sometimes called Madeline a devil. That was Vivian, expressing herself through Madeline, while accepting the mother's label for her. Vivian, who Madeline perceives as classically beautiful, also functions as Madeline's primary sexual part, although all the adult parts can be sexual at times. Vivian is the primary protector of Bunny, the six-year-old. Because Vivian views Bunny as too young to be involved in sexual activities, she ensures that the child is absent whenever Madeline and her husband engage in lovemaking. Like Bunny, Vivian does not view Madeline's mother as her mother, and like Bunny, Vivian views Madeline's father as her father. (Having parts who deny having the same relationships as the outside person is common in the internal world.)

The second adult is Janice. She is the only subpersonality to have developed during Madeline's adulthood. She presents herself internally as plain looking, with no resemblance to Madeline. She does not view Madeline's family members as her own. She first appeared when Madeline was 28 and beginning a new career. The new career was demanding and required a steep learning curve of Madeline. Janice was the part who brought the necessary energy and drive to succeed. She is a worker, an organizer, and a taskmaster, with few interests other than doing what is expected of her. She provides a focus on practical matters while excluding concerns that might interfere with task completion. Domestically, she is also the duty sex part, available to Madeline's husband when Madeline is uninterested in sex.

The third adult is Sally. She was actually the first of Madeline's parts to develop. She first appeared when Madeline was two years old in response to the birth of Madeline's younger brother, the same brother whose death led indirectly to the appearance of Bunny two years later. The new brother was sickly and generally secluded. Sally was anxious about him, reflecting her parents' anxiety about their son's health.

In physical appearance, Sally presents herself as Madeline appeared in her 30s, before she lost weight and toned her body. According to Madeline, Sally says she is roughly 34 years old. She had aged along with Madeline until Vivian, who replaced her as the system manager, became dominant during Madeline's program of diet and exercise a few years previously.

As the system manager, Sally was anxious and depressed. This meant that Madeline was also anxious and depressed. However, as Sally's leadership gave way to that of Vivian, Madeline lost about 60 pounds and became an avid cyclist. Vivian's replacement of Sally as internal manager symbolizes Madeline's shift from an anxious, depression-based view of the world to a positive, action-based view.

With Vivian in control of her internal world, Madeline stayed in a program of physical conditioning, maintained her competence at work, and refused to be submissive in social relationships. Sally, while no longer depressed, continues to amplify negative energy in the form of anxiety. She is a frequent worrier, anxious about the possibility of any significant disruption in Madeline's life. Sally, the worrier, and Janice, the worker, often combine their efforts in order to bring to Madeline's attention whatever problem Sally has seen on the horizon. Sally views Madeline's mother and father as her own.

Four years after Madeline differentiated her internal parts, she described her internal world as stable. She said that because of her awareness of her internal family, her life is fuller and richer now than it ever was before. She felt a sense of being centered and knew exactly what she wanted from life.

In technical language, Madeline achieved *increased integrative functioning* through working with her parts. She frequently consults with her parts now and listens to what they have to say. When she experiences a strong negative emotion, she often seeks out the part who is expressing the emotion so that she can deal with it appropriately.

Madeline does not experience a confusion of identity when a part blends with her. She maintains executive control across all situations. She does not experience "a disruption in the usually integrated functions of consciousness, memory, identity, or perception of the environment," which is characteristic of persons with dissociative disorders.[10] Moments of distress for Madeline are not clinically significant; they are in proportion to the situation. Overall, as the result of her work with Parts Psychology, Madeline continues to experience an enhanced positive functioning.

The Basic Treatment Plan

The procedures for healing through work with the inner world are straightforward. First, find the part that carries the problem behavior, while remaining aware that sometimes more than a single part may be involved. Second, elicit the problem memories held by the part. Third, neutralize the energy attached to the problem memories. Finally, help the now flexible part adjust to a newly defined role when necessary. Sometimes, adjustments have to be made to the basic plan. I describe the most common of these adjustments through the case descriptions that follow this chapter. The following sections sketch the most important elements of the basic treatment plan.

SUD and SUE Scales

In doing Parts Psychology, we will normally collect a set of significant memories from a newly differentiated part, including, whenever possible, its earliest painful memories. These are the memories that must be neutralized if the part is to be flexible enough to change the way it functions. As these memories are collected, it is important to get a sense of how disturbing they are to the patient. The measure to do this is called a *SUD* scale, for "Subjective Units of Disturbance."[11]

The therapist asks the patient to ask the part how disturbing the memory is on a scale from zero to 10, where zero represents neutrality and 10 represents the most disturbing level a memory can reach. For example, a part created to handle the pain of physical punishment might rate its earliest remembered beating as a 10 on the SUD scale, but might rate a later, similar beating as a level 5 on the SUD scale. In working with troubled parts, we want to reduce the disturbances to a zero on the SUD scale.

Sometimes, as with the case of the helper part mentioned above, a different kind of scale is needed because the memories are not disturbing. In such cases, I use a *SUE* scale, for "Subjective Units of Energy." Generally, these memories are positive, but occasionally a patient cannot characterize an event as either positive or negative, just as containing a lot of energy. Thus, a 0-10 SUE scale measures the energy invested in an experience when that energy is *not negative.*

The therapy described in Chapter 4 includes interventions that neutralized the energy attached to a patient's early positive experiences of helping others. The purpose of that therapy was to free the part from its intense desire to please others even to the patient's own detriment.

Locating Parts

Finding a problem part can be easily accomplished by roughly 90 percent of patients. Suppose the problem is excessive anger. I might ask the patient to think about a person or event that causes the patient to become aware of irritation or anger. Next, I would ask the patient to focus on the emotion or its associated body sensations. Then I would ask the patient to speak inwardly to the emotion, asking it "to give you a picture, an internal image of itself." The therapist can increase the probability of the patient locating an image of the part by first coaching the patient to "ask the body sensation to increase its effects" or to "step back" and "step forward" again before requesting the internal image.

The patient can make the request of its internal part while speaking aloud or, as most do, by speaking silently, subvocally, to the emotion or sensation. In the great majority of cases, there is an immediate response and the patient notices an internal image of the part. The most frequent response is an image of the patient as viewed in present time, sometimes dressed as she is in the therapy room, but more often with a different set of clothing, and perhaps with an expression on her face that is consistent with the emotional state with which we are working, e.g., a frown.

Another frequent response is an image of the patient at an earlier age, ranging from a few years younger to a picture from childhood. Less frequently, the patient will visualize a person with no physical similarity to her at all. Still less frequently, the internal image may be that of an animal, such as a lion or a fox, a cartoon figure, or a symbol such as a triangle or a fog. The particular costume worn by the part, i.e., the image visualized by the patient, is much less important than the content of the part's memories.

A variety of other techniques helps a person to visualize a part. When the direct approach above does not produce a viable image, my favorite next attempt is the following guided imagery. I ask my patient to focus on the experienced emotion or sensation and then to imagine the presence of two harmless fisher-men who hold between them a tightly stretched magi-cal fishing net, magical because it can pass through the body without harm.

I suggest that the patient imagine the fishermen walking past her on either side of her holding the net between them. As they walk past her, the net passes easily through her body, but snags on and wraps around the part (i.e., the negative emotion or body sensation). Then, as the visualized fishermen continue walking past the patient, the net pulls the part out of her body. When she visualizes the part emerging from her body in the net, I suggest that she place it gently into a nearby room, and then look into the room and describe what she sees there. The visualized image is the part we are looking for.

Sometimes, when *freestanding parts* cannot easily be located, it is useful to find them as they appear in significant memories. I call such parts *stuck-in-the-memory parts*. Often, when a patient recalls a memory, she may be able to visualize herself in the memory as if she were standing outside the memory scene rather than experiencing it from within. If so, the therapist can guide the patient in interacting with that stuck-in-the-memory self. It may or may not have additional memories or knowledge of the patient's life beyond the memory scene.

A few patients cannot visualize their subpersonali-ties, but still manage to do excellent parts work. Of these, most connect to their internal parts through body sensations. For example, a male patient experi-enced parts' sensations at various locations in his body. There were parts who spoke from the left, right, and back of his head; another manifested as a sensation between his eyes and yet another from the area of the heart. These sensations appeared to be permanent connections between the patient and his parts, and he communicated with them just as well as those who have internal images upon which to focus.

Still another technique for locating parts builds upon earlier success. Once the patient has developed the skill to maintain an internal dialog with a given part, I might ask this part to assist me in finding others. Suppose, for example, the patient had managed to develop a relationship with a task-oriented worker part, but an anger-carrying part had not yet shown itself. In such a case, if anger was an issue, I might suggest to the patient that he ask the worker part if it knew an angry part. If so, the next step would be to request that the worker part bring the angry part onto the patient's internal screen. If this internal bridging is successful, therapist and patient can then proceed with interviewing the new part in the usual manner.

Unfortunately, not all patients are able to develop and maintain an internal image or other means of consistently connecting with an internal part. I find that perhaps 10 percent of my patients are unable to do parts work of any sort. This does not include those patients who can *do* parts work but choose *not* to do so. For most of these latter patients, talking with an aspect of self as if it were a person raises the fear that they might be mentally ill, or might become so through this work. Although such fears are ground-less, it is better to turn to more traditional helping approaches than to force the parts approach on the unwilling patient.

Orienting Questions: Establishing Communication Flow with Parts

When we first make contact with a part, it may be difficult to develop comfortable communication between patient and part. It is a new experience for both parties and requires a short learning process for each. To ease the participants into interaction, I usually draw from a standard set of questions for coaching the patient in developing a relationship with the part.

Parts sometimes present the illusion that they are speaking to the patient with articulated speech. In other cases, a part will be immobile and whatever information is transferred to the patient from the part comes as a phrase or a completed thought, and sometimes not as speech at all but as a scene requiring interpretation by the patient and the therapist. In time, however, the information transfer between patients and parts becomes more efficient.

Remember that images of parts have no actual organs of speech articulation that work as the physical body organs work. Consequently, it is just as easy to talk to a physical object like a balled fist or a color as it is to an image with moving lips. Here are the questions I usually ask, adjusting them to the part's responses. Therapists should feel free to develop their own introductory questions.

1 Ask the part if it knows who you (the patient) are. Ask for a guess if it is unsure or declines to answer.

2 Ask the part who it is and how it is related to you (the patient).

3 Inform the part that it is a part of you (the patient); then ask if it accepts this. Continue orienting questions regardless of response.

4 Ask the part if it knows your mother, father, brother, sister, spouse, son, daughter, and other relevant persons in your life.

5 Ask the part if it considers your mother, father, etc. to be its own mother, father, etc.

6 Ask the part if it likes your mother, father, etc.

7 Note: it is often helpful to ask the patient to provide an image of the relative in question. Often a part will indicate it knows the person by image rather than name.

8 Ask the part how old it is or how old it feels. In the absence of a precise number, ask the part if it feels like a child, a teenager, or an adult.

9 Ask the part how old it thinks you (the patient) are.

In developing this communication the therapist and patient soon learn that different parts have different relationships with the patient's primary family members than does the patient. Many parts may not even know the patient's primary family members. Very quickly, both therapist and patient learn that the concept of a fully integrated person with all subpersonalities sharing the same relationships and memories is a myth.

Memory Sets

The primary content of a subpersonality is its *memory set*. This set of memories provides the distinctive perspective the part brings to the larger self. Most often, these memories consist of a series of negatively experienced events with a common theme. For example, the theme might be improper favoritism and the memory set might contain all of the experiences that support a patient's view that a parent unduly favored a sibling in childhood. The memory set might also contain memories of teachers favoring another child over the patient, or of an employer promoting a less talented worker ahead of the patient. Typically, other experiences that might cast doubt on the perception of favoritism are either not included in the memory set, or are discounted as exceptions and explained away as special circumstances.

A part's earliest painful memory documents the experience that probably created the part. It deserves special attention. If an intervention aimed at reducing the negative energy carried by the part is to be successful, this earliest memory must be reduced to neutrality. Otherwise, many later memories cannot be successfully desensitized. The earliest memory will continue to amplify its negative energy onto the later ones, preventing their desensitization. Additionally, current life experiences will continue to trigger the early memory and create additional distress in the present.

It is sometimes possible to collect a part's entire set of significant memories, both positive and negative. The part is the judge of what is significant. Sometimes, however, there are too many memories to make the task of recording them practical. In such cases, a representative sample is sufficient, ranging throughout the historical period in which the part actively functioned. In most cases, a relatively small number of memories, five to eight experiences, will capture the essence of a part's role. During the processing of these memories, other memories may spontaneously appear, enabling the part to process its entire memory set as the new memories are swept into the unburdening rituals.

There are a finite number of significant memories in the memory set. Additionally, a group of memories with a similar theme can be represented by a single memory that includes all of the major issues, such as fear, anger, and abandonment that appear repetitively over time. For example, a person may have experienced chronic abuse over many years but the part that encapsulates the abuse memories in its content may include in its memory set only the most painful ones. When the patient processes these more powerful memories, he may not consciously register the processing of the less painful memories. Yet, at the conclusion of work, the less powerful memories do not register distress for the part.

The therapist can sometimes safely elicit the full memory set before processing them. However, my experience suggests that the patient is emotionally safer when the therapist helps her process painful memories as they are elicited. Otherwise, she may be overwhelmed later by those emotions she accessed during the session but did not process to neutrality.

For example, a depressed patient who experienced the loss of both parents during childhood might experience a deeper depression in the following days if the therapist does not help her to deal with her unresolved grief before ending the session. Similarly, a man whose extreme anger is fueled by his memories of physical abuse throughout childhood should work through major abuse memories as they appear in session rather than wait until the next therapy session. Otherwise, he may find himself overreacting to minor provocations for the next few days.

A useful guide to working with these volatile cases is to collect only the number of memories that can be successfully processed during the same session. In those cases where it proves impossible to complete the processing of painful memories prior to ending the session, the therapist should help the patient place the unresolved material in temporary storage until the following session. I describe techniques for doing so in the text. One example would be to coach the patient to visualize the part placing its unresolved negative emotions into a safe until next session.

Keeping in mind these cautions, there can be benefits to working with the entire memory set. When therapist and patient together examine the full content of a part's memory set, they can more easily see what should be neutralized and what should be left untouched. Selective neutralization is invaluable for work with certain kinds of problems. For example, many men with pornography addictions have a part that includes within its memory set both normal sexual encounters and problematic pornographic encounters. In such cases, the therapist would want to desensitize the pornographic memories while leaving intact the energies of sexual memories that are not a problem for the patient.

The Affect Bridge

In locating a part's earliest memory, it is sometimes sufficient simply to coach the patient to ask the part to recall it. At other times, however, the part's recall may be aided through an *affect bridge,* a technique developed by John Watkins which, with its companion *somatic bridge,* is widely utilized in Watkins and Watkins' Ego State therapy.[12] With this technique, the therapist asks the patient to speak to the part they are working with and to ask it to connect to the emotion it feels when they discuss a current issue. Then, let the part's mind search back across time for the earliest memory that somehow connects to the emotion it feels in the present.

The therapist might also ask for a somatic bridge by asking the patient to focus on a body sensation, such as tightness in the chest, a knot in the stomach, etc., and search for the earliest memory of that sensation. These techniques do not always reach the earliest relevant memory but the memories that are located are always significant. The therapist may repeat the request using the last memory located and, with that as an anchor, bridge to still earlier memories. I use both of these techniques frequently in doing Parts Psychology.

Unburdening

Unburdening is a technique developed by Richard C. Schwartz,[13] which enables internal parts to discard the accumulated loads of distress they have acquired in their history of protecting the self. The content of a part's burden consists primarily of negative energies such as guilt, fear, humiliation, anger, sadness, etc. that are attached to its accumulated memories. A part is unburdened of these noxious emotions as the therapist guides the patient in working with his internal parts. In working with parts, the Parts Psychology therapist emphasizes that unburdening results from neutralizing autobiographical memories.

The tools for unburdening are visualization and imagination. The patient visualizes the part giving up its burden through some sort of symbolic action. Once the part agrees to relinquish its burden, the therapist might ask the patient whether the part would like to give it up to wind, water, fire, or something else.[14] Depending upon the part's response, the patient might visualize wind blowing the burden away, water dissolving it, or fire burning it up. Other symbolic actions that parts have chosen include throwing the burden over a cliff, flushing it down the toilet, burying it in a deep hole, and using various means of smashing it into nothingness. Once unburdened, the part becomes flexible and centered while giving up its extreme beliefs and behaviors. The patient can now move forward with more positive integrated functioning.

I illustrate below three metaphors for unburdening. The precise language for any given intervention will vary according to the context. These examples address negative emotions, but the procedure is the same when addressing positive emotions that require neutralization. Sometimes the patient will listen and repeat the words to the subpersonality and sometimes he will simply allow my words to pass through to the subpersonality. Occasionally, when my patient has difficulty in reproducing the language or imagery, I will intentionally speak directly to the subpersonality.

•Visualize the part standing in a waterfall and notice how sometimes there are drops of water and sometimes mist and sometimes a powerful pouring of water. Let the water flow over, around and through her. Notice how the part's hair is plastered to her head and her clothes stick to her skin. Ask her to locate where it is within her that she stores the problem memory and then ask her to feel the water dissolving the pain and negative emotions connected to the memory. Notice how the negative emotions dissolve in the water as the water washes them out of her. You may even notice how the water around her is discolored as the dissolved negative emotions are washed away. As the water continues to wash away her anger [or fear, sadness, etc.] you may notice how it gradually becomes clear again as the memory is washed clean.

•Visualize a bonfire for the part and ask him to stand in front of it. Then ask him to locate where it is within him that he stores the painful memories. Now ask him to reach inside of himself and lift out the negative emotions [or negative energy] and throw them into the fire. As the fire touches them, you can see them burst into flame. Ask him to go back for more and keep repeating the action until all of the negative emotions and sensations that were attached to the memories are entirely con-sumed in the fire.

•Visualize the part standing in an open field and bring up a powerful wind to blow over, around, and through her. Ask her to locate where it is within her that she stores the memory and ask her to feel the wind scouring the memories and washing them clean of fear and anger [or sadness, shame, etc.]. As the wind breaks up the fear and anger into tiny particles, you may notice that as the wind blows away from her it is darker because it is blowing away the particles of those emotions like dust or sand. Let the wind continue to blow until the memory is just a neutral memory with no particular emotion attached to it.

Using guided imagery is not new in psychotherapy. What is new is the use of these techniques in a context where subpersonalities are explicitly recognized. The therapist focuses the intervention on an internal part with whom the patient maintains contact as opposed to asking the patient to experience directly the imagined wind, water, fire, etc. The powerful results of unburdening are the direct consequence of working with the specific subpersonality that actually carries the painful emotions in its memory set. A therapist may achieve some limited success through working just with the patient without a direct connection to an internal part. However, the work with internal parts is the source of the dramatic results I describe in this book.

Much of the time, the initial intervention does not fully unburden the part, although the part may communicate that the visualization was successful. This is where the therapist makes use of the SUD and

SUE scales. The therapist coaches the observing self (i.e., the patient) to ask the part how disturbing the targeted experience is now on the 0-10 SUD scale. If we are working with positive emotion, the therapist asks for a measure of the remaining energy on the SUE scale. Typically, the initial unburdening intervention succeeds in reducing the level of distress from, for example, 10 to 6, 8 to 5, or 7 to 2. Repetition of the intervention leads to additional unburdening.

After the initial unburdening, the therapist coaches the patient to ask the part what is the most disturbing aspect of the remaining burden. The unburdening then focuses specifically on that disturbing element. Suppose, for instance, that we were trying to unburden the part who carried the disappointment of a mother's lack of attention while growing up. Assuming that the initial intervention reduced the SUD level to a 3, we might then ask what made it a 3 rather than a zero. The response might be, "Because it's wrong!" We could then ask the part to focus on that wrongness as we repeated the unburdening metaphor. The intervention might require three or four repetitions before the unburdening is complete.

A good example of unburdening positive energy using a SUE scale comes from a case of marriage counseling. My patient, the wife, wanted to hurt a romantic rival in some way. She stalked her around the city for hours. She had twice verbally confronted her. The rival obtained a restraining order against my patient to keep her at a safe distance. Unfortunately, my patient's jealous and vengeful part, overwhelmed by powerful emotions, led her to continue stalking the other woman anyway.

Because my patient recognized that she was putting herself in danger of further legal problems, she agreed to work with her inner world. In working with the vengeful part, we discovered that she acquired her earliest memory at her fourth birthday party, where she received a sandbox as one of her birthday gifts. A neighborhood boy insisted upon "messing with" her sandbox in spite of her demands that he stay out of it. Finally, exasperated, she hit the boy in the head with a rock. He ran home, bleeding and crying.

As my patient relates the incident, she got in trouble for injuring the boy, but she got her sandbox to herself. For the vengeful part, this experience was satisfying to a SUE level of 10. It seems that just as she viewed the sandbox as her property and did not want to share it, she also viewed her husband as her property and was unwilling to share him. In a single intervention of unburdening, however, she was able to reduce the energy level of the sandbox memory to zero. She accomplished this through the symbolic action of visualizing the part detaching the positive energy from the memory and throwing it into a fire. The consequence was that she was able to stop stalking her rival. Later, there were a few other positive memories that required unburdening, but the procedure was the same.

Generally, there are just two reasons for why a part cannot unburden itself completely. First, a manager part, especially an angry part, might believe that it needs the negative energy amplified by a burdened part to fuel its own drive. It fears that if the first part is unburdened, it will not be able to carry out its agenda.

The second reason is the presence of another part, usually a younger one with an earlier memory, who is amplifying its pain to the degree that the targeted part is experiencing the pain as its own. In either case, the task is to find the blocking part, develop a cooperative relationship with it, and then either unburden it or gain its permission to continue the work with the first part. The focus of therapy then returns to the original part in distress.

Unburdening may also stall when the part feels it has not yet been sufficiently heard or understood. The patient may report something like, "She [the part] wants you to know it wasn't her fault." In such cases, it is helpful to halt the direct attempts to unburden the problem emotions and to take time just to listen to the part's story. Once a part has told its story, it is usually ready to return to the work of direct unburdening.

Other Interventions

Unburdening is the most dramatic intervention for bringing about immediate therapeutic change. There are a few other interventions that are also useful at times. For example, listening to a part's story, mentioned above, helps to reduce the negative energy attached to a part's memory set. Such narrative processing of life events is one aspect of nearly all psychotherapies.

What is new here is that the therapist coaches the patient to elicit the narrative directly from the sub-personality that carries the memories. There is something about this direct connection between part and patient that increases its ability to release negative energies as the part tells its story.

Another intervention, one with a long and venerable history, involves changing the way the patient remembers a traumatic event. This sort of intervention can be traced to the 19th century work of Pierre Janet who succeeded in healing distressed patients through revisiting the original trauma memory during hypnosis and changing the remembered outcome with hypnotic suggestion.[15]

In Parts Psychology, similar but less dramatic memory interventions can be helpful in the healing process, but without the use of formal hypnosis. For example, a child part visualized by the patient as trapped in the memory of her parents fighting can sometimes be encouraged to tell her parents to stop the fighting and go to their rooms. If the child part is unable to act in this way, the patient can imagine herself going into the remembered scene to demand an end to the fighting. Finally, if neither the child part nor the patient can imagine herself standing up to the parents, the therapist can ask the patient to visualize the therapist going into the scene and bringing about appropriate changes.[16]

Another patient, dealing with the effects of childhood physical abuse, might imagine his adult self entering the remembered scene of a severe beating and ordering the abuser to cease his or her activity. The result of such interventions can be the immediate reduction, or even cessation, of distress for the part still trapped in the painful scene. For the patient it means that current events will no longer trigger the targeted memory. That memory will then no longer amplify emotional pain into the life of the patient.

Another way to work with traumatic memories is to remove the part from the memory scene. In most cases, this results in an immediate diminution in the part's distress. Carrying out the intervention can be quite simple. The therapist could suggest that the patient visualize taking the part's hand and stepping out of the scene and into another, more comfortable scene. For this purpose, the patient can create an internal safe place, perhaps a combination of a playroom and family room for both child and adult parts. While such a safe place is imaginary to the patient, it is real to internal parts, as is the relief parts feel when going there.

Still another valuable intervention brings about a dialog between polarized subpersonalities. For example, one part may push the patient to take a stronger stand with real world adversaries, while a second part argues that greater success will come from a gentler approach. The result for the patient can be a vacillation between positions, never knowing what is best, with a resultant anxiety over decisions previously made and a dread of making future decisions. An example could be the pressures felt when friends or relatives make unreasonable requests of the patient.

In such cases, the therapist can help to bring about a reduction in anxiety and self-blame by brokering an exchange of views between the extreme parts. Once the patient visualizes the opposing parts, she can encourage them to understand each other's position and to work together as a team for the welfare of the patient.

Parts often take extreme positions because they are afraid that if they give in to the other part, all will be lost and the patient will be damaged in some permanent way. By encouraging a dialog between parts, the patient can bring about a cooperative working relationship between formerly polarized parts, combining the skills of both subpersonalities. The patient thus acquires greater flexibility in the outside world, drawing upon the resources of either part, depending upon what will work best in a particular situation.

Normal and Abnormal

One possible criticism of Parts Psychology might be that the inner worlds of subpersonalities illustrated throughout this book are abnormal worlds, and the persons whose stories are told here could be suffering from dissociative identity disorder or lesser degrees of dissociative problems. In dissociative identity disorder, painful memories are separated (dissociated) from the observing self and sequestered within the boundaries of alter personalities who have the ability to switch into control of the patient for varying periods of time. When such powerful alter personalities take control, the patient typically has no memory for what transpires during the period of control. The presence of these subpersonalities is the most well-known aspect of dissociative identity disorder.

It is one major purpose of this book, however, to argue that having subpersonalities is not abnormal. What is abnormal is the autonomous ability of some subpersonalities to take full control of the person and to leave the observing self with amnesia when the part gives up its control. It is not abnormal, however, for subpersonalities to influence a person from within and thus bring about shifts in moods and attitudes. This is normal functioning.

In order to assure readers that the case descriptions that follow this chapter are descriptions of dissociatively normal people, I have taken pains to choose for this book, with the exception of Chapter 13, only those patients whose scores are less than average on the Dissociative Experiences Scale, the most widely used measure of dissociation.

The Dissociative Experiences Scale

The Dissociative Experiences Scale (DES) is a 28-item questionnaire that measures the degree of dissociation a person experiences in everyday life.[17] Dissociation includes common experiences such as losing track of time and place while driving, or having your mind wander while someone is talking to you. It also refers to more problematic symptoms, such as having the sense that you are observing yourself from outside your body, or having the sense that the world is not real.

Dissociation also includes the separation of painful memories from the person and the sequestering of them in the memory sets of the alter personalities found in dissociative identity disorder. This process may leave the person with few memories of certain significant life events.

Although the dissociation of painful memories into alter personalities is best known in dissociative identity disorder, the process is not in itself pathological. It fact, it is the normal process by which people put aside their problematic experiences and resume normal activities. This may occur, for example, after a death in the family or a disappointment at school or work.

Such memories are collected in the memory sets of normal parts (subpersonalities). Dissociation is the process that brings about new subpersonalities, whether in the normal person or in the case of dissociative identity disorder. New parts form whenever the new experiences are sufficiently novel or too painful for handling by existing parts. The difference between normal and abnormal dissociation lies in the degree of amnesia. With dissociative identity disorder, it may be impossible to access dissociated memories without an alter personality taking control of the person. However, the normal person can generally gain access to partially dissociated memories through concentration and discussion.

The average DES score is 10.[18] Persons diagnosed with posttraumatic stress disorder typically score in the high teens or 20s. More severe dissociative disorders, including dissociative identity disorder, become increasingly likely as scores approach 30 and higher.[19] With one exception, I have intentionally limited the case descriptions in this book to persons who score the average or less than the average of 10 on the DES scale. My intent is to ensure that the case descriptions represent people with normal degrees of dissociation. Thus, the ability to go inside and work with subpersonalities is a normal ability and not an abnormal one. I do not include any cases of patients with dissociative disorders. At the beginning of the description of each case study, I include the DES score of the person in the study.

Endnotes to Part 2

1 Noricks, J. (1981). A Tuvalu dictionary: Volume 1, volume 2. New Haven: Human Relations Area Files Press; Noricks, J. (1981). The meaning of Niutao *fakavalevale* (crazy) behavior: A Polynesian theory of mental disorder. Pacific Studies, 5, 19-33; Noricks, J. (1985). Native-speaker componential models: A method for elicitation. *Ethnology*, 24, 57-76.
2 For example, Noricks, J. (1983). Unrestricted cognatic descent and corporateness in Niutao, a Polynesian island of Tuvalu. *American Ethnologist, 10*, 571-584; Noricks, J. (1987). Testing for cognitive validity: Componential analysis and the question of extensions. *American Anthropologist, 89*, 424-438; Noricks, J., et. al. (1987). Age, abstract thinking, and the American concept of person. *American Anthropologist*, 89, 667-675.
3 Prince, M. (1925). The problem of personality: How many selves have we? *Pedagogical Seminary and Journal of Genetic Psychology*, 32, 266-292.
4 American Psychiatric Association (1994). *Diagnostic and statistical manual of mental disorders (4th ed.)*. Washington, DC: American Psychiatric Press.
5 Roberto Assagioli, the Italian psychiatrist whose *Psychosynthesis* framework is internationally recognized, also developed his ideas in the early 20th century. He called parts *subpersonalities*. See Assagioli, R. (1965). *Psychosynthesis: A manual of principles and techniques*. New York, NY: Penguin Books.
6 Watkins, J.G. & Watkins, H.H. (1997). *Ego states: Theory and therapy*. New York: WW Norton.

7 Schwartz, R.C. (1995). *Internal Family Systems therapy*. New York, NY: Guilford Press.

8 For example, see Stone, H. & Winkelman, S. (1989). *Embracing ourselves: The voice dialogue manual.* Mill Valley, CA: Nataraj Publishing. The authors interpret parts (subpersonalities) as the local representations of Carl Jung's archetypes.

9 Helen Watkins describes an intervention she calls *the silent abreaction,* which has some similarity to the unburdening concept. However, it appears to apply only to the release of anger. See: Watkins, H.H. (1980). The silent abreaction. *International Journal of clinical and experimental hypnosis, XXVIII,* 101-113.

10 American Psychiatric Association (1994). *Diagnostic and statistical manual of mental disorders (4th ed.).* Washington DC: American Psychiatric Press.

11 Wolpe, J. (1990). *The practice of behavior therapy (4th ed.).* New York, NY: Pergamon Press. In bringing the SUD and SUE scales to Parts Psychology, I was influenced by Francine Shapiro's use of the SUD scale in her EMDR treatment model. See Shapiro, F. (2001). *Eye Movement Desensitization and Reprocessing: Basic principles, protocols, and procedures. Second edition.* New York, NY: The Guilford Press.

12 Watkins, J.G. (1971). The affect bridge: A hypnoanalytic technique. *International Journal of Clinical and Experimental Hypnosis, 19,* 21-27. For the somatic bridge, see Watkins, J.G., (1992). *Hypnoanalytic techniques: Clinical hypnosis (Vol. 2).* New York, NY: Irvington.

13 Schwartz, R.C. (1995). *Internal Family Systems therapy*. New York, NY: Guilford Press.

14 Schwartz, R.C. (2005). *Freeing the Self: Releasing the exiles.* Workshop presented 01/01/05-01-07/05, Esalen Institute, Big Sur, California 93920.
15 Ellenberger, H.F. (1970). The discovery of the unconscious. The history and evolution of dynamic psychiatry. New York, NY: BasicBooks.
16 Asking the patient to visualize the therapist intervening in the memory scene is a favored technique in ego state therapy. See Watkins, J.G. & Watkins, H.H. (1997). *Ego states: Theory and therapy.* New York, NY: WW Norton.
17 Bernstein, B. & Putnam, F.B. (1986). Development, reliability and validity of a dissociation scale. *Journal of Nervous and Mental Disease, 175,* 727-735.
18 Putnam, F.B. (1997). *Dissociation in children and adolescents.* New York, NY: Guilford Press.
19 Putnam, F.B. (1989). Diagnosis and treatment of multiple personality disorder. New York, NY: Guilford Press.

About the Author

Jay Noricks originally trained as an anthropologist, getting his PhD in Psychological Anthropology at the University of Pennsylvania. His fieldwork on the island of Niutao in what is now the nation of Tuvalu provided the data for his PhD dissertation. The 15 months of study in Tuvalu also led to the publication of a Tuvalu-English, English-Tuvalu dictionary and a series of papers in cross-cultural cognition. The first of these papers was "The meaning of *fakavalevale* ("crazy") behavior in Niutao: A Polynesian theory of mental disorder," published in *Pacific Studies*.

After many years of university teaching as a professor of anthropology, Jay changed careers to begin clinical work in psychotherapy. He established a private practice in psychotherapy in 1996 in Las Vegas, Nevada.

In 2011, Jay published his book, *Parts Psychology: A trauma-based, self-state therapy for emotional healing* (Los Angeles: New University Press LLC). He has conducted training workshops in the practice of Parts Psychology since 2007 in Morgantown, West Virginia; Denver, Colorado; and Las Vegas, Nevada. Currently, he writes, maintains a private practice in psychotherapy, and conducts workshops from a base in Las Vegas, Nevada.

Other books by Jay Noricks

Parts Psychology: A trauma-based, self-state therapy for emotional healing

A Tuvalu dictionary. Two volumes: Tuvalu-English, English-Tuvalu

Made in the USA
Middletown, DE
10 November 2021

the Timberline Review

ISSUE 11 | 2022

A publication of Willamette Writers

Editor-in-Chief	Maren Bradley Anderson
Executive Director	Kate Ristau
Associate Editor-in-Chief	Louise Cary Barden
Fiction Editor	Rankin Johnson
Poetry Editor	Suzy Harris
Nonfiction Editor	Manny Frishberg
Script Editor	Grant Rosenberg
Art Editors	Jan Baross
	Kathleen Caprario
Copyeditors	Angela Celeste Atkinson
	Michael Colvin
Proofreader	Jaime Dunkle
Readers	Ella Ananeva
	Jason Arias
	Tina Brazeau
	Linda Caradine
	Ellen Kozyra Currier
	Morgan Grey
	Kathy Haynes
	Asela Lee Kemper
	Stephanie Striffler
Cover Design	Lee Moyer
Interior Design	Vinnie Kinsella, Indigo: Editing, Design, and More

Editorial Correspondence: http://timberlinereview.com/contact/

ISBN Print 978-1-7320427-9-7
ISBN eBook 979-8-9864222-0-6

DEDICATION

Thank you to the Willamette Writers Board of Directors for continuing to trust me with *the Timberline Review*. The staff of this journal is entirely made up of volunteers, including the editor-in-chief position. If you like what you see here and want to know how it is done, consider joining Willamette Writers and volunteering to work on the next issue of *the Timberline Review*.

CONTENTS

TRANSFORMATION

Letter from the Editor

When we chose "Transformation" as our theme for this issue, we wanted artists to explore life in flux. We hoped they would consider their world transformed; we anticipated that they would examine hope and possibility and change. We thought perhaps they would look into the future and help us settle the past.

This theme made me think of butterflies like the ones on the cover of this issue. The butterflies I imagined were born of wretchedness, but were being transformed into other-worldly, impossible beings that would transcend the horror of what happened to them in their chrysalises.

I thought that visual representation of change would be a metaphor for what we've all been through in the last several years. But I know now that my personal transformation has not made me a lighter-than-air being.

Although the sun has finally ended an unusually long, wet, and gloomy spring here in the Pacific Northwest, I still feel like one of those dark butterflies—gothic and floating, but not at all "light." I feel like a creature made of stained glass, whose brittle wings are fashioned of lead barely connecting fragile panes of color, and a filament holding me above a windowsill.

And I know I am not alone. Writers and artists answered our original challenge with essays and fiction about the instants when lives change, scripts about pivotal moments, poems and pictures about shifts in perceptions. Lightning literally strikes in these pages, children grow, and visitors appear at the edge of the world. People are missed, and missions are discovered.

Sometimes the works in this volume are very dark, and sometimes they glow with love. Yet, every piece reminds us that life is hardly static.

During the process of transformation, we may not understand what we will become, but we can feel the ache of our wings and perhaps the pull of the filament keeping us aloft.

Maren Bradley Anderson, Editor-in-Chief, July 2022

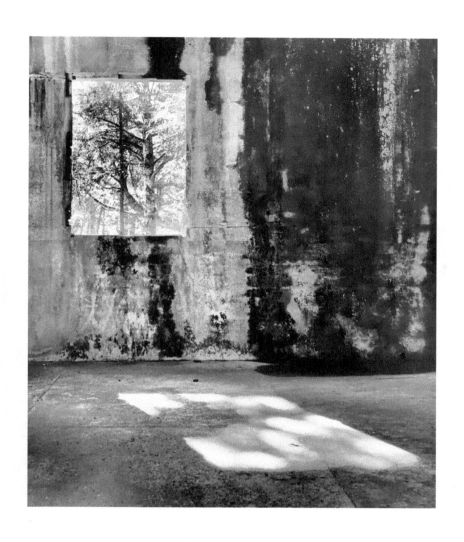

THE VIEW IS BETTER
Photograph by Kitt Patten

THE ASTRONOMER HAS WINGS

Poem by Keli Osborn

E pur si muove. (And yet it moves.)
—attributed to Galileo

Moons of Jupiter, phases of Venus, shifting specks
on the sun. Illusions in his primitive scope,
the devil's work. And the priests refused to look.

    Waving in the winds, monarchs turn in winter
    to the cypress, eucalyptus of California, Oyamel fir
    of Mexico's mountains. The fourth generation wings

    between home and home, swarms unfamiliar trees
    in a singular encounter. Ordinary miracles fill the air
    with a hum, wonders could stagger the certain.

The astronomer wore heresy through fever, unto death.
Circling a star, earth spins mutation. Caterpillars remember
how to create the silk button, tuck into chrysalis and wait.

EVERY INTERACTION I'VE HAD WITH THE MOON

Poem by Colette Tennant

leaves me flirtier somehow.
I mean look—that coquette of a
peek-a-boo moon,
that heartbreaker, that tease,
twirling her wispy skirts
over the silvery mountains east of here.

Every interaction I've had with the moon
makes me an optimist again,
amazed by her sideways smile—
how it dwindles, disappears, then
grows so bright it emblazons
even November nights.

Every interaction I've had with the moon
reminds me: we mothers,
we're always watching,
leaning down our faces over those we love,
humming our honeyed songs
into the sweet, bluesy dark.

FLOWERS OF UNUSUAL ORIGIN
(OR A SELECTIVE INVESTIGATION OF THE CAUSES AND EFFECTS OF KERAUNOGRAPHIC MARKINGS UPON A TEENAGE FEMALE SUBJECT)

Fiction by Claire Alongi

Mrs. Bean's *Understanding Biology* Summer Assignment:

A key aspect of our class this coming year will be using our powers of observation to gain a better understanding of the world around us. This summer, I want you to pick something that you view as a common or essential piece of your life and, over a seven-to-ten-day period, observe and analyze it in the way a scientist would. You could examine your family dynamic, the way your soccer team behaves, or maybe even where your cat goes when it leaves the house. The possibilities are endless, but be creative! Look for details, ask questions, draw connections, and try to understand this thing in a new way. Do further research if you come across something interesting. Keep a log of your observations which can be turned into me on the first day of class. I hope you all have a wonderful summer and good luck!

Observations Log:
Days in house: 1
Days since incident: 4
Current time: 02:41

The Subject has not brushed her hair, washed her face, or taken a shower since returning. She was escorted into the house by The Father at approximately 14:30, and since entering her room has not left. To my knowledge, she has not yet removed her hospital band. In the brief time I was able to observe her, she appeared stiff and tired, jerky in movement.

Her eyes were strangely still and distant. Her hair was limp and flat with grease, and the bags beneath her eyes were so dark they seemed painted on. The walk from the driveway, past the kitchen, through the family room and down the hall—which normally The Subject would accomplish at a sprint, especially given her propensity to flee from and avoid annoying boyfriends, The Father, and the agitated younger sibling among others,—was negotiated at a slow shuffle with frequent stops.

The Father looked too old. Despite the early gray in his curls, and the sadness everyone knew he hid, there always seemed to be a youthfulness in his loose movements, in his quickness to appreciate bad puns and bathroom humor. If The Subject had not been in her current state, I suspect she would have made a playful jab about his haggard appearance. As it was, both parties moved slowly, silently, to The Subject's room.

The Father and I dined alone without The Subject. It was takeout from a family-owned Mexican restaurant six blocks away. The Father ordered our favorites: a #2 combo with two shrimp tacos and two steak tacos for him, and for me a rice and bean burrito—no salsa, sour cream, or guacamole.

"How was your day?" The Father asked.

I shrugged and told him it was uneventful.

The Father proceeded to tear off small bits of tortilla and nibble them slowly.

"Your sister is still pretty…out of it," he said.

I told him I knew.

"Recovery time for this is really varied," he said.

I told him okay.

"I know you were young when Mom… When what happened to Mom… Your sister saw someone then, though. A professional. If you want to talk to me or someone else about what happened with your sister that's more than okay. I know it was scary. I was scared. It's okay to feel that way."

I chewed slowly and deliberately and shook my head while counting the grains of rice that had fallen from the burrito onto the placemat.

For sake of scientific accuracy, I feel obliged to report that there were four pieces of rice lying on the woven blue of the mat. I swallowed my mouthful of chewed burrito.

I told him I was fine. I was fine then, and I was fine now. I knew it was okay to be scared, but I wasn't scared. I was fine.

He sighed and rubbed a hand over his face.

"Okay. You can change your mind," he said.

We put our leftovers in the fridge. Neither of us had eaten much. I walked past The Subject's room. She lay completely still and straight on her back, arms neatly settled over the top of her quilt, eyes closed as she breathed softly. The Subject typically nests—contorting and manipulating her bed covers into a kind of cocoon. To see her sleeping so rigidly was unnerving, almost like The Father had brought back a quiet, unobtrusive changeling.

Days in house: 3
Days since incident: 6
Current time: 01:13

The Father will return to work tomorrow at The Subject's insistence. He is not pleased, but The Subject has become slightly less lethargic and insists that having him hover over her will not help her recover. At breakfast she pointed her fork at me, mouth still full of scrambled eggs, and said, "Plus, Dad, she's not totally useless, right? There's a reason you have a back-up child—it's for things like this." As she said it she looked at me with a muted version of her toothful smile as if to say *you know I'm just joking right*? It was a familiar expression, a familiar joke, but it seemed foreign on her still washed-out face. The Father offered a short, strained chuckle nonetheless.

Although The Subject has not left the house since her return, she is fond of sitting in front of windows. I suspect that, after several days in the fluorescent maze of the hospital, she craves sunlight. Yesterday afternoon, she dragged a collection of blankets, pillows, and stuffed animals from her bedroom to the family room and sat herself against the coffee table facing the sliding glass door to the backyard. She's moved little since then, only occasionally switching between her book and laptop. She, of course, relocated as necessary to utilize the bathroom, for lunch and dinner, and to return to her room to sleep.

Both The Father and The Subject went to bed long before me. But several hours later when I was brushing my teeth in the bathroom, I heard some shuffling and emerged to find The Subject again situated in her spot by the coffee table.

When she saw me peeking my head from the bathroom door, she said, "Come here, there's something I want to show you." I sat down next to her in the pile of blankets. She had finally, and thankfully, showered right before bed and smelled of her lavender shampoo and hibiscus body wash. Her hair was no longer gross and shiny, and even though she still seemed vaguely waxy and skeletal, she was less like the walking corpse she had been a couple of days earlier.

"Look at this," she said, and pulled her left arm from underneath a quilt. "They're called Lichtenberg figures," she said, tracing an intricate branching pattern that seemed branded into her flesh. The marks reminded me of the skeletons of a leaf, or maybe a feather. They started out mid-forearm and ran all the way up to her shoulder before disappearing in the sleeve of her nightshirt. "My doctor said that they're created by the pattern of ruptured vessels from the strike," she said, then continued on almost wistfully, "Probably will be gone in a few days. Kinda sad they're not going to last. They're a bit badass, right?"

NOTE: Lichtenberg figures were first observed in 1777 by a German physicist named Georg Christoph Lichtenberg. He found that airborne dust settling on electrically charged plates created branching tree-like patterns. When found on lightning strike victims, they are also called lightning flowers, though the medical term is "keraunographic markings."

I nodded my affirmation. The Subject was pleased and wrapped herself back up in the blankets. She stared out the glass door and into the yard where moonlight was illuminating the overgrown grass and abandoned tree swing. Without looking at me she said, "Did you know that the weather report didn't call for thunderstorms that day? We were supposed to be in a little dry spell. I probably would have skipped the run if I'd known. It came out of nowhere. I cut across the soccer field to get home quicker when I got hit. I wonder if I'd just come home the normal way if it still would have happened," she said, then paused for a moment. "Do you think it was supposed to happen? Like fate maybe?"

The Subject is not typically this philosophical, and generally pokes fun at people (e.g., her younger sister) for entertaining even mildly deep or grandiose musings. I told her that fate wasn't involved, that she definitely wasn't to blame, that it was just really bad luck. I asked her why she was out of bed, why she wanted to tell me these things, but when she didn't respond, I looked over and saw she had fallen back asleep, her body awkwardly slumped against the hard edge of the coffee table, her neck lolling forward onto her chest. I maneuvered her down, so she was lying on the rug. She didn't wake up, and I wondered if she had been truly awake during our conversation. The last time The Subject sleepwalked, to my knowledge, she was seven or eight years old. She woke me to say that there was something coming, something that was going to make us all disappear just like Mom. She told me we needed to leave right away. I grabbed Bunny from my bed and stumbled out into the hallway, past The Subject, terrified that I would be the last vanish. That there would be a brief moment when I was all alone. Before I got far, The Father scooped me into his arms. He sang to me as he carried me back into my room. In my panic, I hadn't even noticed that The Subject had fallen asleep in my bed. Gently, The Father scooted her to one side and somehow all three of us managed to squeeze into my tiny bed. We slept soundly the rest of the night until morning. And we were all still there when I woke up.

NOTE: According to Met Office, a British weather think tank, there are approximately 1,400,000,000 lightning strikes per year. Lake Maracaibo in Venezuela receives more lightning strikes than any place else on earth. During massive storms, it may receive as many as 40,000 strikes in a single night. The National Geographic website says that about 2000 people die each year from lightning. "Hundreds more survive strikes but suffer from a variety of lasting symptoms, including memory loss, dizziness, weakness, numbness, and other life-altering ailments. Strikes can cause cardiac arrest and severe burns, but 9 of every 10 people survive. The average American has about a 1 in 5,000 chance of being struck by lightning during a lifetime."

Most people survive lightning strikes, I learned, because the lightning often doesn't actually hit them directly. There's this phenomenon called "flashover" where lightning zips over the body (in as quickly as three milliseconds) via sweat and rainwater. Metal objects can be hot enough to burn, and shoes and socks can be thrown from the body.

The Subject was found by two neighbors who lived next to the soccer field and saw the strike. They performed life-saving CPR on The Subject until the paramedics arrived and are heroes in this observer's estimation. Her running shoes and wicking socks were scattered ten feet from her body. Though I have not seen it, apparently, she has a burn in the shape of our house key at the small of her back from where it was zipped in her running shorts pocket.

Days in house: 6
Days since incident: 9
Current time: 23:37

There was a knock at the door twenty minutes after The Father left for work. Still donning her rumpled terrycloth robe and mismatched fuzzy socks, The Subject untangled herself from her coffee table nest, and moved quickly to answer it. While not yet at full sprint, she managed a decent fast walk even with the slipping of socks on the hardwood. At the door stood a couple of very confused men. One stared skeptically at The Subject, while the other seemed to be assessing the house.

"We're here from the LEC? We thought this was some kind of business… Did you order?"

"Yes, yes I did order the spline ball ionizers," The Subject said before he could finish.

The man didn't seem convinced.

"Listen, is there an adult here?"

"I am an adult," The Subject said with authority, narrowing her eyes. The man seemed a little nervous then. "I'm an adult, and I can pay," she said, producing her wallet from some pocket within the robe. Then, for the first time since she had returned from the hospital, The Subject stepped out of the house. She hesitated on the front porch for a moment and, almost imperceptibly, glanced upwards at the clear summer-blue sky before walking towards the van parked in the driveway. The men turned to follow her as if she was now their leader. I lingered in the front door.

The logo on the van's side panel featured a large golden lightning bolt inside a bright red circle with a diagonal line through it. LIGHTING ELIMINATORS was printed in that same bright red just to the right of the image. The Subject stood and watched in her robe and fuzzy socks as the two men began unloading equipment from the back of the van.

The man who seemed to be in charge turned to her and said, "Listen, normally we install these things on big commercial buildings and huge metal structures, ya know?"

"I ordered them, and I want them installed," The Subject said. The man shrugged.

"Whatever, it's your money," he said.

Over the next few hours I puttered about inside the house while The Subject watched outside as the men climbed onto the roof and put up whatever it was they were putting up. I could hear their thumping footfalls overhead. Finally, the sound stopped, and I heard the van pulling out of the driveway. I joined The Subject on the front lawn. I asked her what the *fuck* the things on our roof were. (Sorry Mrs. Bean; I'm recording for accuracy.)

"They're spline ball ionizers. They help prevent lightning from striking. I don't totally get how they work. Something with lowering the electrical current, grounding point, I don't know," she said.

NOTE: According to the Lightning Eliminators & Consultants website, "the patented [Spline Ball Ionizer] SBI is a hybrid lightning protection concept engineered to provide multiple levels of protection for critical applications. In its primary mode, the SBI lowers the risk of direct strikes by utilizing a phenomenon known as charge transfer, where a well-grounded point exchanges ions between the air and earth. This ionizing capability helps keep the local electric field below lightning potential, making the protected site less likely to experience direct strikes."

The spline balls looked like metal dandelion puffs attached to slender flexible poles; they waved just barely with the breeze. There were three of them poking up from different points on our roof. To be fair, they weren't enormous, but they were far from inconspicuous. I told The Subject that The Father was going to kill her.

"Nah, he can't say anything. And if he does, I'll just remind him that I was actually clinically dead for like five minutes." I couldn't help myself, I told her that, without question, she was definitely going to die again. (At that point, she called me a name I cannot repeat, Mrs. Bean, even for accuracy.) Then she walked back into the house.

I remained on the lawn, thinking about how nine days ago I was an only child for five minutes, around the length of a long song. It occurred to me that there could well come a time when I'd again be an only child, but likely not before I become an orphan. It's a thought I'd never allowed myself to have fully formed, but I think it had been lurking below the surface of my thoughts for a while, maybe longer than I'd like to admit. I shoved it back under, though it didn't go willingly.

A chill went through me, and then I followed her indoors.

NOTE: Emotional lability, sometimes called emotional incontinence or psuedobulbar effect (PSB), is a neurological condition that can lead to inappropriate, exaggerated, and uncontrollable outbursts of laughing or crying. This, according to the Healthline website. "While the symptoms of emotional lability seem psychological, they're actually a result of changes to the part of your brain that's responsible for emotional control."

Days in the house: 7
Days since incident: 10
Current time: 01:21

The Father was, indeed, not pleased by the spline balls. He was home late on the night of their installation, but this morning he was in full fighting mode. So was The Subject. I stayed in my room while they tore into each other.

"Jesus Christ, we can't afford those things," he said. "Call the company. Have them come back." The Father was using his End of Discussion voice.

"They're for protection," she said.

Both their voices were getting louder.

"We don't need protection from lightning! What happened was freakish bad luck! You were just in the wrong place at the wrong time" he said.

"That's exactly what you said about Mom!"

This was a shriek.

"Pea…Sweetheart…You know what happened to Mom was a very different thing."

This was soft.

"But I died too, Dad! I WAS FUCKING DEAD!" My sister was sobbing. And then, abrupt silence.

I suddenly became aware that I was holding every muscle in my body at attention, but even with that knowledge, I couldn't bring myself to relax. Distantly, there was the echo of another moment long ago and mostly forgotten, of a cold house, emptier than normal, police officers hovering, my father quietly weeping at the table while my sister clutched me to her chest, her tears in my hair.

But now instead of crying there was laughter. My sister was laughing.

I cracked open my door and looked down the hallway towards the kitchen where they were standing on either side of the table.

"I'm sorry," she gasped through hiccupping guffaws, "I don't know why… I'm laughing?" But she didn't stop. And though she still laughed, tears pricked at the corners of her eyes. She laughed like I'd never seen her laugh, doubled over, convulsing, her breath coming in short gasps. Dad rushed to her. He folded her into himself and stroked her back while she trembled so hard they both fell to their knees. Finally, her fit subsided. My sister's eyes, though, were wide and afraid.

"The doctors said things like that might happen. Your brain is just trying to sort things out still," Dad reassured. Wordlessly, she extricated herself from his embrace, picked herself up from the floor, and drifted towards her room. She closed her door slowly, softly, as if it might break. He stared after her without noticing the sliver of my teary face peeking through the small opening of my door.

My Dad let out a deep sigh and sat down at the table with his head in his hands.

"Fuck," he said flatly. "Fuck."

Days in the house: 10
Days since incident: 13
Current time: 23:19

Backlit by the moon on a clear summer evening, the spline balls swayed in the night air like colossal, fabricated, lightning flowers. My dad, my sister, and I stood on the lawn and watched them. No one knew quite what to say, so for a while, we stood in silence. It wasn't exactly comfortable, but it wasn't quite awkward either. After a while my dad shuffled back inside after giving each of our shoulders a gentle squeeze.

"I think they're growing on him," my sister said quietly, voice rough from the laughing and crying that still came and went seemingly without cause, building and shattering the tension in the house, leaving us strung out. Changed. But we'd been rearranged before, from four to three. We could do it again, move with the volatile electrical current of our lives, I hoped.

And if not, at least tonight we could pretend.

I nodded my affirmation. Her smile was still softer, more distant, and I realized that it might not ever quite return to full wattage.

"You're staring at me," she said.

It's nothing, I told her. Everything is fine.

The corners of her lips inched up just a bit more. For a moment we just looked at each other. The tension broke when she turned and began to walk towards the house.

"The spline balls will protect us," she said as way of parting, spinning around briefly before disappearing inside.

I couldn't tell if she was saying it to convince herself or me.

Either way, I wanted to believe her.

GROUNDED

Poem by Kate Maxwell

Under a dripping tap
he washes his pointy head
    sleek coal feathers
greased and gleaming
in the hot afternoon sun.

Crow hops crookedly
across the park, a creaky
old man, too long on horse
    bum high and awkward
as his slimy feathers leak.

Hurling cranky squawks
at round-eyed pigeons
pecking in the dirt, *Caw! Caw!*
    his half-raised wings
craning neck, a fisted threat.

Fat bobbing birds scatter
from his Darth Vader cloak
let him rule until dog-time
    when sudden flight
    fills the sky, black sheen

of his elliptical extravagance
spreads broad across
    a cobalt canvas
    and the grounded
    become glorious again.

A LONG WAY FROM HOME

Poem by David Mihalyov

The western sky appeared
in western New York today,
dimming the sun, seeding
the clouds, replenishing
our soil with the remnants
of trees burning thousands
of miles away, our rain
unfamiliar to the memory
of smoke that traveled
over the Rockies, the Plains,
the rust belt, a reverse
manifest destiny ending south
of Lake Ontario, the green
and softness as strange
to those particles as the walls
of flame and DNA of Ponderosa pines
are to the sugar maples
and paper birch we walk among.

DEEPEST LIGHT

Fiction by Sandra Siegienski

The alien ship appeared in our cloudless blue Australian sky one day, a silver disc settling above the ocean a hundred kilometers offshore, making contact with no one. Ships approached, but ocean waves consistently diverted them away. Planes attempted flyovers, but winds set them off course. Soon, the military arrived to investigate.

"Who are they, Daddy?" my five-year-old daughter whispered. Her wide brown eyes, so like her mother's, stared at the disc's image on my laptop screen.

I wondered why Serena was whispering. "I don't know, sweetheart. But I'm hoping they've come in friendship."

"They haven't said hello."

"Maybe we need to say hello first."

She thought about this, her little chin propped on her hand. "How do we do that?"

"We're trying all kinds of ways." Signals of every kind had been sent, but so far no one had received a response. The ship hovered near the coastline where our cottage sat above the seaside cliffs. Although I'd dreamed of interstellar connections, I realized that I found such close alien proximity disquieting. Serena kept running to the window to try to see the craft, though, all eagerness and bouncy curiosity, so I tried not to let my worries affect her.

Washing dinner dishes, I listened to both newscasts and an abundance of speculation. The birds that usually rustled in our eucalyptus trees had grown unnaturally still, long before nightfall. I kept a close eye on the yard while Serena played on the back porch in the waning afternoon.

When sunset came, Serena and I cuddled together in my easy chair, watching the brilliant colors of the sky change.

"They still haven't said hello." Serena wiggled around, searching for the ship one more time.

"Maybe tomorrow."

"Are they scary?"

"I don't know." I wanted to reassure her, yet not give her false words. "So far, they seem to be patiently waiting. Maybe they're curious and listening to us. The best way to get to know someone is by listening. They might not speak our language. Maybe they're deciding what to say." I wanted to believe my own words. The ship might not be in sight, but I felt its presence anyway.

Serena didn't answer. She stared at the ocean, making me picture a young rabbit in a grassy meadow, waiting.

"Why do *you* think they're here?" I asked her, curious.

She rested her head against my shoulder. "I think they want to get to know us." Her voice sounded unnaturally hollow.

A chill settled in my stomach, and I held Serena closer.

The blue hour came and went. We fell asleep curled up together. I awoke to stars shining in a clear sky. Serena lay awake, gazing at me. She seemed to be looking through me.

"What, sweetie?" I sat up, unnerved.

"I think they're trying to discover things."

It took me a second to remember the ship. I glanced at the window. "That's quite likely." Serena's discerning expression was not one that a child five years old should have. I'd never seen that look on her face before.

"It's bedtime." She lifted her arms up to me.

I picked her up. She wrapped her arms and legs around me, clasping my shirt, resting her face against the soft cream-and-green plaid that my wife, Mia, had given me last Christmas, when we'd thought we'd have so many more years together. "I'll tuck you in."

"I had funny dreams."

Her flat tone didn't sound like her. "Dreams about what?" With a sinking feeling, I carried her up the creaking stairs, wondering where this was going.

"Someone was talking to me."

My hair rose. "Did you understand them?" I kept my voice even, hoping she wouldn't feel my heart starting to pound.

She sighed. "No. But they kept trying."

I reached the top of the stairs. A crayoned picture of a sky with bright yellow sunshine hung taped to the door of her room, reminding me of the spring when Mia and I had taught her how to color. Serena loved sunrises, and her drawings were filled with suns and swathes of pinks and orange over shoals of fish.

After bath time, I carried Serena to her bed, settled her in, and told her favorite bedtime story about little koala bears and bunnies and pots of golden honey. She clutched the coverlet her mother had made—before last year's tragic car accident had taken Mia from us. Serena's fingers seemed so small against that bright, intricately pieced quilt. I wrapped its comforting softness around both of us.

"Will the ship be here all night?" Serena asked, hushed. "The birds like it being here."

We hadn't heard their song for hours. "I think it'll be here for a while. It came a long way." I chose my words carefully, but I couldn't suppress a little shiver.

"We'll be okay, Daddy." Serena patted my hand.

What do I say? "I think you're right, sweetheart." I gave her a kiss and tucked her favorite stuffed bear under the covers, so it lay nestled against her. Only last week, Serena had said that she was five years old and had outgrown sleeping with teddy bears.

Tonight, she did not object to her bear. She clasped it under her arm.

I added, "The ship's people might like learning, like you and I do—" I tickled her belly and she giggled "—and maybe we'll learn some new things, too."

She nodded sagely. "Learning is crucial. Understanding is essential."

A chill went down my spine. Serena never spoke this way. She'd voiced moments of childhood wisdom that delighted me, but nothing like this. I closed my eyes. When I regarded my dear daughter again, the light in her innocent eyes had changed slightly, that clear sweetness shining of joy and discoveries, all suffused with my wife's twinkle of humor.

I took Serena into my arms and kissed her again, wishing with all my heart that I could protect her on this strange new journey we seemed to be beginning.

Serena gripped my thumb, something she hadn't done since she was three years old. She closed her eyes, curling up to sleep.

I stayed in her room until dawn, vigilant, reading on my phone all the reports about the ship, researching its effects, while watching Serena shift and mumble in her sleep. Did we need help? Whom should I contact, and what would I tell them?

Saturday.

Serena and I watched broadcasts about the ship, played outside a little—until the heat nudged us indoors—and took naps on the sofa, where three of us used to sit together, not just two. Serena woke often, seeming to listen to sounds I couldn't hear, but she said little. Her gaze roved constantly over things she'd seen many times. My paintings—many landscapes, still lifes, and portraits covering our walls—particularly drew her interest.

Birdsong returned to our trees, but the birds were departing. Great flocks and migrations of all species had begun shifting in the ship's direction. Huge shoals of fish had begun moving that way as well, along with pods of dolphins and whales. Naturalists and biologists were alternately intrigued and growing alarmed.

The public's reactions ranged from curious to increasingly fearful. Unrest was growing in the cities. I was glad we lived away from town, away from any frenzied panickers. I still couldn't decide what to do, or whom to contact about Serena. Instinct told me *wait, just wait*. I tried hard to listen.

Scientists and the military started capturing affected wildlife for study. I pictured them capturing Serena. I could find no reports of children being affected, but that didn't mean it wasn't happening. I picked up my phone a dozen times but couldn't force myself to call anyone. What if someone took my Serena away to study her? What if someone took my beloved child, so soon after I'd lost Mia?

Would I endanger her more by trying to protect her myself? I didn't want to remove her from the safety and security of her own home. What if whatever was affecting her simply followed us? Home, and all its familiarity, seemed the safest place to stay.

Serena had little to say that evening. On the sofa, she curled up in my lap, having wrapped herself up in her fluffy yellow blanket, a favorite of her mother's. My heart ached. Again, the image of a little rabbit came unbidden to my mind.

I spent the night in Serena's room, watching as she tossed and turned in her sleep.

Around midnight, I awoke to Serena shaking my shoulder. She stood beside me, dressed in her green-and-white fuzzy pajamas, her little feet in fuzzy green slippers, clutching her blanket around her like a halo. "They're talking to me, Daddy," she whispered, shaking my shoulder again. "I don't understand them, and I want to go back to sleep."

I rose and took her in my arms, unsure if I was fully awake and half-hoping I wasn't. The expression in Serena's eyes scared me—their light was changing. A quiet calm and deep perception now filled them. My daughter was no longer fully herself. Someone was speaking to her, through her. "Use me, instead. Leave her alone!" I called to no one. "She isn't the one you should choose!" Then, I worried and chased my fears, pacing the floor, until my head ached.

A long day later, the ship remained offshore, with the whole world focused on its presence.

Serena sat on our tiled kitchen floor, surrounded by sheets of paper, holding a fat red crayon in her restless little fingers, drawing circles and lines and discs and grids, like timeless watch pieces filled with splintering gears and mechanisms.

"What are you drawing, honey?" I kept my voice steady, despite outright fear mixed with wonder, struggling to keep my calm, to *wait…wait….*

She looked up, her sweet brown eyes all innocence, and yet filled with wisdom that shouldn't belong to her so soon. "It's a story, Grandpa."

A story? "I'm your Daddy, honey," I told her gently. "Grandpa is—"

"You look like Grandpa." She stared at the family photo on the wall, between my paintings of Mia, then dropped her gaze back to her fevered drawing. "I can see him in your eyes."

I thought of how many times Mia had told me I resembled my father. *You have his eyes*, she'd said. Hearing those words from Serena gave me shivers.

"What kind of story are you drawing?" I quickly asked, pointing to her sketches. "Are these like the pictures I draw for picture books?"

She stopped drawing for a moment. Her gaze did not leave her pages. "It's a story about our future."

Serena's random crayoned elements became pictures. Gears became clocks. Clocks became advanced mechanisms that I no longer recognized.

My daughter, the light of my world, of all my being, was growing further and further from me. I couldn't bear to watch her disappear. I researched endlessly—everything from telepathy to sonic communication to possession. Publicly, wild theories abounded about the ship. It still ignored all communication attempts. People were deserting nearby towns. Roads were becoming jammed.

Birds kept flocking to the ship, and fish kept congregating. Was someone communicating with them? Perhaps if I'd shared my wife's aboriginal heritage, I could have shared her understanding of dreams and the earth and its complex connections. I needed that wisdom. Serena was sharing something with our visitors, who stayed just out of my reach.

I tried to contact Mia's elderly aunt, but transmissions were disrupted.

Again, I considered packing up and leaving, but I couldn't risk losing Serena by abandoning the safety of home. I was afraid, and I didn't like it. I dreaded the darkness of night because sleep brought me no comfort and brought my daughter only dreams that weren't dreams, through which she kept drifting further away from me. Every new, unfamiliar expression on Serena's face scared me more.

As much as I'd longed to contact alien races, I'd never expected it to be like this.

On the fourth day, I brought Serena outside for the sunrise—a father-and-daughter time we often shared with mugs of hot chocolate filled with whipped cream. I'd forgotten our tradition during the past few days.

At first sight of the rising sun-diamond, Serena covered her eyes. "It's too bright, Daddy!" she cried. "Make it stop! Make it go away!"

With tears in my eyes, I gathered her up against my chest, covering her eyes, her head—anything to shut out whatever was tormenting her—and headed for the house.

"It's the sunrise, honey. You've seen it so many times." I didn't feel my reassurance myself. What was it about our human eyes that our visitors didn't understand yet? They must have seen so many suns and stars.

"But it hurts." She whimpered until we reached our house's calm darkness. There, we sat in Mia's beloved rocking chair, and I rocked her. Serena quieted, murmuring, "The brilliance is astonishing."

What do I say? "Don't look straight at it, darling. Our eyes can't do that. It's always been bright like that." But I wondered, *where are we going next?*

If only I could understand this transformation, instead of fearing it. Could I guide our visitors to what they might wish to learn? Anything for Serena.

Rose and gold clouds filled the sky after sunset as I walked Serena through our local park, telling her about koalas, wallabies, forests, and the land's history, as if it were all new. Serena clutched my hand, studying everything intently as if seeing it for the first time. The sweet scent of eucalyptus, Mia's favorite, enveloped us.

As the sky grew dusky blue, Serena pointed out a young man sitting on a boulder, holding a long tube of wood. "What's that?"

"A didgeridoo," I told her. She regarded it with deep interest. I led her toward the musician. I'd tried learning to play a didgeridoo before she was born. It took skill. "You blow into it a certain way and it makes sounds."

The young man smiled at her and began playing a deep, intricate melody and rhythm while I admired his abilities.

Serena listened, intrigued. "Can you play all the notes at once, Daddy?"

"No, honey. You play one at a time."

She considered this information in silence. "I think you're wrong, Daddy." She pulled me away to a traditional Japanese wooden bridge arching over a dry waterway.

"A didgeridoo isn't designed to be played that way," I said. But then, it wasn't my native tradition, so I couldn't really speak with any authority.

"There are many designs with which you are not familiar." Serena explored the bridge's construction intently.

I couldn't argue. How many designs would we be learning? Would one of them help me get my little girl back? I said, "Please. Will you show me some of these designs? And I will show you some of ours."

After another restless night, Serena sat watching me from her blue chair at the breakfast table. Her place faced away from the windows, and I kept the blinds closed against the sun. To me, the house felt smothered by the shades, but she seemed comfortable. I took a box of eggs from the fridge, hearing on the news that sea turtles were gathering around the ship, alongside the multitude of whales and dolphins.

"Why?" Serena asked, puzzled.

"Why what?" I cracked open an egg and dropped it into the heated pan. Eggs like sunrises—*medama yaki* in Japanese, I recalled—eggs cooked so they look like eyes gazing at you. It had always seemed funny. Mia and I had so often cooked eggs this way.

Whose eyes were looking at me today?

"When you look at me, you're always questioning," Serena said.

I paused in my egg-cooking, oh so careful. "That's because you ask surprising questions. I never quite know what you're going to say, and I want to have the right answers for you."

She nodded, her eyes deeply thoughtful, like no five-year-old's eyes should be. "You like teaching."

"Yes." *But I've never taught like this.* "I like teaching everyone who wishes to learn. I teach whatever I can."

After cleaning up breakfast, I found Serena lying on her bedroom floor, drawing and coloring with my colored pencils. Although she'd often watched me use them to make sketches for my paintings, she'd never requested them before. I sat down beside her. The papers spread across the floor were filled with complex diagrams, designs, and architectural masterpieces.

I swallowed. "Can you tell me about these, sweetie?"

She glanced up, her gaze lasting a few seconds too long. "It's a story for you, for later. They're learning much from us."

"Why do you use paper instead of other methods?" How far had she traveled from me, and who was seeing our world, our home, and our life through her eyes?

"I enjoy your archaic method." Her gaze returned to her designs.

"The symbols are pleasing to the eye."

"Most symbolic representations are," she said, patting Mia's quilt, "owing to the complexity therein."

With love mixed with fear, I studied my little daughter. *Will you come back to me, Serena? When we've learned enough?*

She pushed a piece of paper toward me, her child hands too small to be manipulating the knowledge they held. "You draw too, Daddy."

I paused, selecting an orange pencil, Mia's favorite color. *The color of joy.* The ever-present deep ache in my heart expanded, and I longed for her loving, supportive presence. "What should I draw?"

Serena tilted her head, considering. "Draw life."

I held the pencil above the paper for a long time, envisioning Mia, our daughter, and our quiet home by the ocean. A place of such beauty and love. When I completed my drawing, Serena studied it at length, focusing on the images of our family, then gazed across the house, as if seeing once again into the future.

Evening.

Serena sat in my lap with her yellow blanket, as I was watching-but-not-watching a few minutes of the latest news about the ship, which was still attracting sea and avian life in massive numbers. Even land mammals had begun drifting eastward in this new, strange migration. Environmentalists were growing frantic.

I couldn't concentrate on the information. All I could think about was my own little creature nestled in my arms.

Today, Serena had covered the walls of my studio with minute sketches of buildings and ships—designs which in all my years as an artist I'd never conceived of.

"The ship is going away tonight." She clutched this evening's bedtime book—her favorite story about the tree that gave.

I held my breath for a second. "Is that so?" I kept my voice neutral. *Will it take you with it? Take you away from me?* "Where is it going?" I never wanted Serena to leave my arms again. I couldn't imagine life without my daughter, my joy, my memory of Mia.

"Away," Serena whispered. "They've learned what they desired to learn."

"I hope they've learned many good things. Many helpful things."

She considered this. "Yes. Many things. Speaking our languages. Knowing what the fish say and what the birds sing. Hearing what the land and the people say and don't say."

"I'd like you to stay and listen to the fish with me." I wished it with all my heart, but who would be in my arms in the morning?

"Daddy."

Serena shook my arm, her worried face close to mine, her sable hair rumpled from sleep. "You were up all night in your chair!"

"Yes." I sat up, shaking the haze of sleep from my mind. Sunrise peeked through the blinds in tentative beams. The tone of the news broadcasts had changed—wonder , excitement, relief, and loss. I grasped Serena's hand, trying to comprehend what the newscasters were saying.

The ship.

Gone.

I stared down at my Serena. My little girl gazed back at me, her innocent brown eyes wide. Her own light shone in them, clear and deep and true, with a twinkle of Mia's humor and a faint hint of new wisdom.

"Is that you, Serena?" I took her face in my hands, my voice quaking.

She held up for me a portrait of my wife, drawn with my colored pencils, capturing a beloved moment on the day Serena was born. Mia was cradling our child, while I held both of my loved ones in my arms. "Someone drew this!"

I took the picture with trembling hands. Someone had understood.

Serena giggled, the same bell-like laugh she'd made since she was three years old, the joy of Mia's and my days. "Of course, it's me, Daddy. Who else would I be?"

PRUNES

Poem by Michael Hanner

On a day best spent getting lost
on some empty, sun-dappled French road;
cranking through the gears, downshifting
into the shady curves in our rental Renault,
I'm cleaning out the refrigerator in the *gite*
where we and friends have idled away September.

Now in early October someone's fig jam
and someone's black cherry preserves
are left behind with a few of Cecelia's carrots
still surviving in the vegetable bin.
Nearby several different bowls of olives,
Toni and Linda bought, wait now
on the drain board, fated for the black *poubelle*.
The milk goes down the drain.

Lastly, three sticky bags of succulent prunes
from markets the width of *Périgord*.
At least half remain after pork with prunes
and chicken breasts with prunes and eating prunes
for snacks and eating prunes while driving
on curvy empty, twisty roads, some sun-dappled,
some cloaked in deep plum-colored shade.

SOME SENSE OF IT

Poem by Nancy Nowak

I caught a scent, hint
of the sun's warmth
on the light air
turning like the path
toward spring

held onto now
only in words
retold while we take in
the burnt breath of
early autumn, Ponderosa pine
surrounding the High Desert

rest area. In a breezeway
display panels interpret
what lies ahead
with a map, what we might meet
in these woods

captured in nighttime
images: lucent eyes alert, bobcat and bear
sniff the air, grasp at the dark

as we might try
to shape and keep what is
already changing.

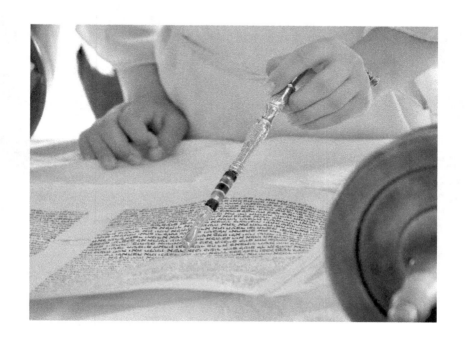

THE MOMENT OF BECOMING AN ADULT
Photograph by Kitt Patten

YOUR MUSIC

Poem by Melody Wilson

—for Stacy

I must have been eleven when I
    tipped you over, tickled your belly

as you dangled down the bedside. You
    a toddler in soggy Pampers, delicate

throat stretched taut; an instrument created for
    this single note—a giggle so dry,

so breathless, I already knew I would never
    hear it again. I was too young

to be in charge while your mother worked,
    pumped gas for the man she thought

loved her, not the first to hurt you, not
    the last. He cast you into the future,

like dice. You called it *free spirit*, but there are
    other words: victim, addicted,

all the tricky gates between toddler and teen,
    teen and woman. You never questioned

the story in the mirror. *The pretty girl*, you always
    said, to describe yourself, voice a reed

between laughter and loss. *The pretty girl* in the
    homeless camp, in the web of friends

you spun. Today the mirror breaks. It no longer
    holds you, and neither does the world. Someone

will close a narrow door, turn a dial. I will step outside
    all these miles away and listen as you flood

into atmosphere: traffic, wind, November leaves
    settling on the lawn, all of it—all of it

following one instant of pure delight, chin thrust
    forward, the perfect laugh of a child.

WALKING TRAIL IN CUNNINGHAM PARK

Poem by Joyce Schmid

A skinny path, concrete,
a city kind of trail with slender trees
on either side all leaning sideways
in a choreography of change.

The New York air was clean
and apple-sweet, the antidote
to cigarette smoke in the close
apartment where my mother lay

in conversation with the dead.
The creaking of the trees seduced me:
ten more steps, just ten more steps,
ten more. Around the bend—

a dogwood turning autumn-red
just like the one in our backyard.
But this tree burned and glowed,
a miracle of morning fire

that would not be consumed—
a sign—
the sea would part
and let my mother through.

SKIN MEMORY

Poem by Margaret Chula

Today I am reading my mother's letters,
written on onionskin, her penmanship tracking
her descent into illegibility, words spilling
down the page and into marginalia.

I read them aloud. Breathe her alive on this day
of smoky skies and windless trees. Make offerings
of blackberries from the brambles, rosehips
bright in my palm, green tea in a porcelain cup.

Porcelain skin, a gift from my thin-skinned mother,
hiding her bruises under long-sleeved blouses—
scribbling her pain in letters full of cross outs
and tear stains.

I am looking at calendars from her final years,
where she noted every phone call—birthdays
of her seven siblings, children, and friends
marked with their birth and death dates.

For the last three months before her death
the calendar squares are empty—numbers
crossed out, as if she were counting down
the days before she would be released.

Somewhere in my skin memory,
we're together again, embracing
beneath a blue sky. And hovering
just above us, a hummingbird—

the blur of its paper-thin wings.

THINGS I WILL NEVER DO

Nonfiction by Caitlin Diehl

You and I will never travel to Hilton Head in a September, after school starts and the crowds are gone, exploring the South Carolina lowlands, scouting for eastern birds we've never seen before, walking with fingers curled together along an empty beach at low tide.

We'll never travel to New England in the fall to see the glorious colors of the season's change, never comment to one another that Oregon is just as beautiful, if not more so, and why did we come all this way for something we have at home. We'll never hike the Blue Hills, you patiently identifying for me every unfamiliar plant and bird, rarely needing to consult the many guidebooks stuffed into your daypack. I won't be able to buy real maple syrup and fresh apples at a farm stand along a country road, offering you the first, crisp bite as I wipe the juice off your lips with the back of my wrist.

Old England is out of our reach as well, though I still hope to go there someday with our daughter, Grace. She and I will be much more compatible travelers than you and I. We would giggle at the same cute Englishmen at the table next to us in the little café around the corner from our hotel where we'd drink pots of tea every afternoon after a late start to the day, and cross off most of the items, still unseen, on our ambitious touring list. You would want me to rise early and get a jump on the day, the list of historical sites laid out before us like mileposts on a marathon course, me game, but tired before we even started. We'd both like the Lake District, though I couldn't keep up with your long legs tramping over the wet fields: you scanning the terrain like an expedition scout compiling a report for his commanding officer; me dreaming of scones with clotted cream and yet another pot of hot tea, happy to be with you while seeing Europe for the first time. Yes, it would have been my first time in Europe, which you would jokingly lord over me, regaling me with stories from your family trip back in high school, undertaken as a cure-all after your sister's attempted suicide. We both know the backstory but don't mention it, focusing instead on the good memories of your first experience out of the U.S., and the "castles you have known."

You would not have wanted to go to Ireland, though our daughter is just as keen as I to see the green land of my ancestors. She is not motivated so much by love of family history as she is a love of dark-haired, blue-eyed boys with accents. Still, all three of us would hate the smoky pubs no matter how good the local fiddler and her band.

What I miss most now is the chance to tear up together at Grace's wedding, you with graying temples walking her proudly down the aisle, telling her pre-wedding stories about the day she was born and how you held her for the first time, alone and terrified, while I slept off the drugs from the C-section. I won't get to press your hand and lean my head against your shoulder as she recites her wedding vows to a man both of us have concurred privately we're not sure is good enough for her.

When I turn 60, seven Julys from now, with my dear girlfriends by my side, out at a Salem restaurant not currently imagined by its future owners, I'll laugh at the bawdy cards while drinking a glass of pinot noir. My friends and I will exchange news of our kids—tales of first jobs won and lost, grad school, a marriage or maybe two—none of which you lived to see, the future a curve in the road beginning just beyond your last breath.

I can't know for sure those hoped-for experiences would have become memories if only the cancer hadn't cut short your life. But I had dreams about our unfolding future with our daughter off at college: you and I growing older, you bemoaning your decreasing running mileage, me my increasing pounds; decades of conversation, of travel, of small hurts and deeper wounds, healed and forgiven. All these are lost to me, as you are lost. Our shared path through the woods, illuminated by our joy in life and in each other, has ended. Now it's all I can do to feel my way careful step by careful step over uncertain terrain through the unending dark.

IN THE POTTER'S STUDIO

Poem by Glenn Vecchione

He works the pedal in erratic rhythms
like a bus driver braking some snare of highway
or Redbone, in shaded rapture, stepping his high-hat
through a syncopation.

But the potter's work is more important
as it powers the wheel beneath the hands
which create the pot of the lump from the Earth
and that's something of a miracle.

His foot creaks under the rods
that wave like a spider doing calisthenics
and set the spin of the discus above
in a pure crucible of creation

but for the jitter of its lopsided orbit
around this orifice of clay—now widening to gape
now pursing tight like a mouth, the potter
aware that each catch in his rotor smears

a ridge, nicks the glisten of this perfect form
but must be allowed, just as the growing numbness
in his hands must be allowed
although it keeps him from throwing more pots

to pay for fuel. He'll be cold this winter
without her and she'll be warm with another
whom she chose because he had money and a hard-
fired thrust and he fell short in both those areas.

This throw reminds him: the pot rising
and thinning like an ascendent pipe of coral,
the species that thrives on morsels and exerts
little effort, the species that continues to grow

until it falls to pieces quietly without complaints.
He too was born open to the world and sturdy,
but low to the ground. Now the keening gyre
of the starry all-surround has ground him thin

but brought him up higher where, observant but frail,
he thrives on whatever comes—even the numbness
of hands because they're still his hands as he throws
this pot under his solid roof on the cusp of October,

the field-pumpkins burning like lanterns in the dusk,
and on his stove another pot where a fine chili bubbles,
the snow gathering distantly over some mountain
whose name he can no longer remember.

THE NAMING

Poem by Lucinda Trew

I should have named him taro
the eldest, taproot from which
all otherness stems and sprawls
like earthen veins, the rhizome
of origin, bloom and stalk

I should have named him in dirt
ear to the ground, attending
for breath and tremor, the echo
of ancestors whispering
his name from burial mounds

I should have covered him with loam
tucked shell and nail and Solomon's
seal around flinty bed, a lock of hair
and holly wing, witches' charms
and arms deep in clay, tilling ground

to tend the graft and splice
of this new life, I should have nursed
him with marrow, compost of bone
and ash and the lore of those
who came and named before

I WOULD HAVE STAYED

Fiction by Natalie Dale

As I step across the threshold, the smell crashes into me. Mildew, dust, and old urine mixed with something else. Something dark. Something dead. I don't want to go in, don't want to face whatever horrible surprises he's left for me. But if I don't, he wins.

The hardwood floor creaks and buckles as I step into the foyer. In my memory, these floors were immaculately clean, washed and waxed until they shone. But now they're scratched and worn, the planks so rotten I worry they'll give way beneath me. It's hot in here, the air thick and cloying. When I told Sofia, the executor, that I wanted to come in alone, she seemed relieved. Now I understand why.

I glance into the living room. It's been twenty-five years since I was here. Nothing has changed, yet everything is different. The plush, pink velvet couch still sits against the back wall, the seat cushions replaced with a wooden plank. The overstuffed red armchairs flanking it have divots so severe that sitting in them would be quite uncomfortable. With Mom's bad hip, rising would have been impossible. I guess that would have been a pretty good metaphor for her reality—uncomfortable, but in too deep.

As I start down the hall, I notice the porcelain dolls crowding every available surface. They stand like sentries on the bookcase, the hutch, even the dining room table. Their unblinking eyes bore into me, and I shiver as I push open the swinging door leading to the kitchen.

My eyes water as the smell intensifies. I pinch my nose shut, but I can still taste the rancid air. A garbage can sits open, flies buzzing dark and thick over the moldy trays of microwave dinners. Dishes—Mom's precious, blue-willow china—sit unwashed in the sink, mounds of moldy food barely visible through the thick covering of flies. On the counter sits the carcass of a dead mouse, its flesh crawling with maggots.

Bile rises at the back of my throat. I turn and flee, out through the overgrown garden and back to my car. I sink to the ground, head in my hands, gasping for air.

A car door opens, then footsteps, a hand on my knee.

"Aww, honey," says the executor, "are you all right?"

I look up, scrub tears from my cheeks with the palm of my hand. Sofia kneels beside me, her forehead furrowed with concern. She isn't much older than I, fifty at best, but she's patting me on the back as if I were a little girl.

"That bastard," I growl. "That fucking bastard. Did you know?"

Sofia takes a deep breath, curls an absent finger around her long blond ponytail.

"Did I know he was leaving you a nightmare? Not exactly. But I was his lawyer for almost a decade. I knew what he was."

I shake my head, run fingers through my newly short hair.

"And I only get my cut if I clean the house up to sell it."

A muscle twitches in Sofia's cheek.

"He made that very clear in his will. You get 50% of the pretax proceeds if, and only if, you clean and prepare the house for sale yourself. If you knock it down, or sell it as-is to a developer, the whole thing goes to charity."

I shake my head. "I'd never knock it down."

Sofia nods, though I can tell she doesn't understand. How could she? She never saw it when my parents lived here together, when the house was full of love and roses.

I turn, frowning at the paint, the gutters overflowing with leaves and debris. Then my gaze lands on the rosebushes filled with deadheads and my stomach sinks. That garden was Mom's pride and joy. For a moment, I'm ten again, racing along the twisting garden path, playing tag with Lisa.

My stomach clenches and I turn away. Everything went wrong after Lisa died. My parents split, and Mom turned to the bottle. I'd thought nothing could be worse than having to drag your drunk mother off the floor, turning her sideways so she didn't drown in her own vomit. But then *he* showed up.

"It'll probably go for half a million," Sofia says, and I'm wrenched back to the present. "It's not huge, but it's in a great neighborhood."

"That much?"

Sofia purses her lips, tilts her head as she examines the house.

"Definitely. If it weren't in such terrible shape, it could go for quite a bit more. Housing prices in this area of Portland have skyrocketed in the past few years."

I bite my lip, try not to pay too much attention to the hope blossoming inside me. I need this money.

"I just wish I could let you hire a cleaner," she continues, her voice full of regret.

I take a deep breath, twist my golden wedding band around my finger. I hadn't spoken to my mother in twenty-five years, not since that horrible night he'd tried to pin himself against me. I'd begged her to run away with me, begged her to leave the man who, despite knowing her for less than a year, had already transferred all her assets into his name. But even then, I knew she'd never leave. He was the one who'd gotten her sober, the one who'd pulled her out of her rock bottom. She threatened to tell him everything, so I left without a backward glance.

"No," I say softly, "I need to do it."

Sofia raises an eyebrow but says nothing. She couldn't know that this was all my fault. That I'd refused to answer my mother's calls, rebuffed my dad's gentle urging to let her apologize. But by the time I graduated high school and was finally ready to talk, she'd stopped reaching out. When I finally got up the courage to call her, I was told by that too-familiar, nasal voice, that she would never speak to me again.

I tackle the gross things first—the mouse carcasses, the dishes, the garbage. As I work, sweat pools in my armpits, beneath my breasts, the insides of my thighs slapping together with every step. Of course,

I'd have to spend the hottest weekend on record cleaning out a house without air conditioning.

Pausing by the pile of garbage bags, I wipe my forehead with the back of my hand. Even with the doors and windows flung open, with candles burning in every room, and the countertops drenched with Clorox, there's a lingering smell.

Him.

According to Sofia, he died of a heart attack and was found by the police weeks later. I imagine him dying alone, rotting like an avocado on the green linoleum floor. The thought makes me smile. I only wish it hadn't been a heart attack. He didn't deserve a quick death.

Next, I pile the dolls into garbage bags. I remember Mom's collection of porcelain dolls, their exotic clothing and silky hair. She wanted one from every country in the world. But this collection is whitewashed: all blond curls and blue eyes; their ruffled dresses pastel variations on a theme. I save one—a black-haired doll in a kimono, the sole survivor of Mom's cultural collection—and donate the rest.

Even with the dolls gone, there is an absurd amount of shit. Useless brick-a-brac line the shelves and plaques filled with clichés like "happiness is homemade" clutter the countertops. Every wall sports collages and framed photos of them and them alone. I scour the kitchen drawers, the bookcases, searching for a memento—something, anything—she'd kept to remind her of me, Lisa, Dad, her parents, or even one of her friends. But there's nothing. No shred of evidence that my mother's world consisted of anyone but him.

The pang of regret is followed quickly by the sharp sting of anger. Mom chose him, chose this life of isolation and alienation over me. And ultimately, it had killed her. She'd died of breast cancer, caught late because he wouldn't let her out of his sight for a mammogram. I didn't learn this from him, naturally, but from her soft-spoken best friend, Becky, with whom she was allowed to speak—chaperoned, of course—once a week. There wasn't even a funeral.

Finally, the house is empty, and I stand before a closed door. I've spent the last week washing windows and cleaning algae-clogged toilets, filling dumpsters and donating carloads to charity. I've hired contractors to repair the floor, as well as roofers and an exterminator. Today is my last day alone in the house. I've put this off for far too long.

I hesitate, hand on the doorknob to my mother's bedroom. I have so many beautiful memories there—cuddling between my parents as they read confusing Japanese poetry, jumping on the bed with Lisa, bringing Mom breakfast on Mother's Day—that I'm afraid to go in. I don't want those memories tarnished.

But the contractors are coming tomorrow. I take a deep breath and turn the knob.

The room is dark, navy-blue blackout curtains falling to the floor, and blessedly cool. There are two twin beds—one neatly made, the other rumpled—hulking in the darkness. I stand in the doorway, light flooding from the hall onto the floorboards, and I feel like I'm about to be sick. Everything that was good about this room—the windows flung open to let in the scent of roses and honeysuckle, the queen-size bed filled with pillows, the beautiful Norwegian quilt passed down from my great-grandmother—is gone. Even the air feels static. Trapped.

Hands shaking, I flip on the light and start pulling things from the walls, tossing them straight into a garbage bag. I open the closet, unceremoniously shoving shirts and pants and dresses into donation bags, then do the same with both nightstands. Her dresser is untouched, her bottles of perfume, lipstick, foundation, and rouge lined up beneath the mirror like tiny soldiers. Even her underwear is neatly rolled in a drawer. Her jewelry box is empty, and I feel a little pang of loss. I would have loved to have one of Mom's beloved brooches, even the stupid little bumblebee pin I painted for her in third grade. But Sofia told me he sold off all her jewelry right after she died.

I donate all her clothes but toss everything of his straight into the garbage. No one else should have to wear his filth. Gritting my teeth, I strip his bed—the unmade one, of course—and throw the bedding in the garbage too. I drag the mattress out to the dumpster and dismantle the bedframe. Finally, there is only one thing left to do.

I walk to my mother's bed and, hesitantly, sit down. The mattress is hard, unyielding. I lie down and press my face into the pillows. And there, for the first time, I sense something of her. It's so faint I'm probably imagining it, but I think I can smell her. The vanilla perfume she always wore, mixed with the faint scent of her Olay moisturizer. I close my eyes, feel the tears burning against the back of my eyelids.

A coldness settles around me, and I sit up, slam a fist into the pillow—once, twice, three times.

"Damnit," I whisper, then louder "damnit!"

I throw the pillow hard against the dresser.

"You didn't have to live like this," I shout. "You had me! You had Dad! You chose this fucking monster over us!"

I stand, yank the covers off the bed, snarling as I stuff them into a donation bag. But as I start to pull the sheets, the mattress slips against the box spring, and something falls to the floor. I hesitate, then kneel and pick it up. It's a piece of paper, ripped from a paperback and wrapped around a photograph.

The photograph is of me and Lisa, our arms thrown around each other's shoulders, hair whipping in the wind, our faces upturned to the sun as we stand on some long-forgotten beach. Beneath, in my mother's beautiful cursive, are two words—*my love.*

I trace the words with a shaking finger, repeating the words over and over in my mind.

My love.

Finally, I turn my attention to the poem. It's a long one, torn from the *Collection of Ten Thousand Leaves*, which Mom used to read to us when we were small. I recognize the first stanza

<u>To a Daughter More Precious than Gems</u>
by Otomo no Sakanoue no Iratsume

Heaven's cold dew has fallen
and thus another season arrives.
Oh, my child living so far away,
do you pine for me as I do for you?

My eyes skim the poem, landing on a single couplet towards the end, which Mom underlined three times.

If I could have prophesied such longing,
I would have stayed with you.

A lump rises in my throat. For the first time in twenty-five years, I begin to understand why she chose this life. It wasn't because she loved him more, or because she was weak. She chose to stay so that I could leave.

I tuck the photo and the poem into my jacket pocket, then turn, leaving the rumpled linens on the floor. I don't look down, don't acknowledge the gleaming hardwood planks that now bear a resemblance to the floors of my childhood, don't linger on the empty shelves or holes in the wall where photographs of my family should hang.

As I walk out the front door and close it tight behind me, I feel the tears sliding hot and wet down my cheeks. Because only now, decades later, do I finally understand the cost of my escape.

FORGIVENESS

Nonfiction by Cristina White

Maybe I forgave you when I was seventeen. No, not really. It was only a kind of silent pact you and I made. We agreed not to be in constant conflict, and I set aside my hate and said all right, we will make our peace, and I will trust you never to hit my mother again.

You died decades ago, and in October, my mother will have been gone from this earth for twenty-two years. There is no end of loving her, of being grateful to her and missing her laughter, her generous ways, the good food she made, her courage and loving kindness. I talk to her often, but I never talk to you, and tonight I think I should talk to you. Maybe we should have it out, because I've heard that carrying anger and hate is a burden, and maybe it is time to let it go. Dear God, I want to let it go before I die. No one knows when that will happen, but it will happen. None of us gets out alive.

The truth is, I don't hate you. I used to when I was young and full of rage and despair and sorrow. I was fifteen and there was an afternoon when I heard you yelling at my mother, and I wanted to kill you. The knife was there. I picked it up and I was ready to drive it into you and make you stop. Stop. Stop. But then you were there in the doorway. You were looking at me with a knife in my hand, and I knew it would not end well. Your six-foot-plus, two-hundred-pound body would have the better of me. The knife would be turned against me, into me.

I set the knife down and walked out of the house. That was the day I knew I had to leave, get away, before one of us maimed or murdered the other. I told my mother I had to leave, and I did leave. My grandmother and I took a bus and traveled nearly 3,000 miles away to live with my brother in California. I was there with my brother and grandmother for over a year, until finally my mother asked me to return. We missed each other too much.

I returned, and it was better then. It was as if a cool, moist wind had dampened the fire-hot air in our household. I remember a day when you and I drove to a spot where the dogwood trees were in full bloom. We walked there, and you said, "Let's bring some of these home to your mother," and we did. We brought white flowering branches home for her, for our home. And that was when I felt we had settled things between us, and I could rest from hating you.

Two years later, you broke my trust again. You were drunk, and you hit my mother. And that was it. I could not forgive you. I could never trust you again. And though my mother was desolate when her marriage was finally over, I was glad you were gone, and grateful when she was herself again and made a life without you.

This was all decades ago, and I am weary of this burden. Tonight, I want to remember the afternoon we walked among the flowering dogwood trees, and there was an hour of peace between us. I think about the legend of the dogwood, and those who say the wood of this tree was used to build the cross—the cross on which Jesus was crucified. It is only a legend, a story told in the Deep South. It is a story I can hold onto because you and I were in the Deep South that afternoon we walked in a grove of dogwood trees.

Tonight, I place myself once more in that hour of countless white blossoms, and I think of Christ, who forgave us all. I say to the night sky, to you, "I forgive you." I remember and thank you for the good you gave me, for the times you reached into the well of a loving father and gave me water to drink. I forgive you your faults and weakness and the torment you bequeathed, this pain and sorrow I have carried for too many years. I lay it down in this sacred ground of forgiveness.

I lay it down that I may rest, and you may rest.

Rest. Peace be.

LEARNING TO RUN AGAIN

Script by Lisa Lee

Time: Morning

Place: A private hospital room

At Rise: JULIA (early 40s) is alone in the room speaking on her BlackBerry.

> JULIA
> This is fucked up, Bill! The trial is tomorrow, and you're raising this defense now for the first time? (Beat.) Well, you know I'll have to ask for a postponement and your client will have to waive a speedy trail. And incidentally, the man was completely coherent when the officers questioned him and that's what they'll testify to.

EVELYN (late 60s) shuffles into the room in her hospital gown wheeling her IV. JULIA rushes to help her.

> JULIA(CONT'D)
> Look, I have to go now but we'll finish this conversation later today. (Hangs up). Mom, why didn't you call me in?

> EVELYN
> I don't need you to wipe my butt.

                    JULIA
Yeah, but you've never had to go to the
bathroom with sedatives going into your
veins.

Julia examines the IV bag.

                    EVELYN
Oh please, it hasn't even started working
yet. The nurse was here five minutes ago.
(Beat.) Was that work?

                    JULIA
The defendant's lawyer says they're
introducing new evidence. I can't really
say much more.

                    EVELYN
Julia, you know that it'll be on the news
in a few hours.

                    JULIA
They're claiming insanity. Now I have
rethink everything.

                    EVELYN
You're a good prosecutor. You'll get that
man.

                    JULIA
Mom, I'm going to be extremely busy
the next few weeks, so I've made some
arrangements. Martha and the ladies will

come to visit you on a rotating basis. And
I'm going to get you a nurse for your first
few weeks of recovery. I'll come as much as
I humanly can.

                    EVELYN
I'll manage fine. I don't need a nurse,
Julia.

                    JULIA
You need someone to help you. When you get
back on your feet, we're going to move you
to Orchard Hills.

                    EVELYN
Oh, Julia, not that again! I *like* where I
live.

                    JULIA
You don't need to be living in such a
big house. And you shouldn't be climbing
stairs in your condition.

                    EVELYN
I'm not going to an old fogey place.

                    JULIA
Everything at this place is geared towards
active seniors.

                    EVELYN
That's a euphemism for "old farts."

                    JULIA
It'll be good for you to be around people
your own age.

                    EVELYN
I have my Bridge Ladies, the neighbors.
I've got plenty of people to hang out with.
Besides, you're the one that needs to be
around people.

                    JULIA
Mom, I don't have time to "hang out."

                    EVELYN
You need to date, Julia. You need to find
yourself a companion. Your beauty will
only last for so long.

                    JULIA
Thanks, Mom. You always have a way with
words.

Julia types on her BlackBerry.

                    EVELYN
Julia, do you think that people who make
amends before they die (beat)...do you
think/ they....

                    JULIA
/What are you talking about?

                    EVELYN
These last few weeks, I've been thinking
about....Well, if I don't survive this
operation, / then...

                    JULIA
/What do you mean, 'if you don't survive'?

                    EVELYN
I could die during the operation.

                    JULIA
Mom. You're getting hip replacement
surgery.

                    EVELYN
Some people don't wake up from the
anesthesia.

                    JULIA
Mom, you're going to live to be ninety
years old, just like Grandma Kate. Is this
why you didn't sleep last night?

Evelyn doesn't answer. JULIA goes back to her
BlackBerry. Pause.

                    EVELYN
Julia, something's been really weighing on
me. I want you to know/ that...

                    JULIA
/Mother, you're not dying.

                    EVELYN
This could be our last conversation, and I
want you/ to...

                     JULIA
/The doctor said that you'll be up and
running around soon.

Julia's BlackBerry buzzes. She reads a message
and responds.

                    EVELYN
They say everything will be alright. But
all they do is confuse me. (Beat.) I never
thought I'd say this, but I wish your father
were here. He'd know exactly what to do.

Julia (stops typing, annoyed)

                     JULIA
Dad was an ophthalmologist, not an
orthopedic surgeon.

                    EVELYN
He'd know what to do in a hospital. He'd
know how to talk to all these doctors. He'd
know what all these tests were.

                     JULIA
He would have been a total asshole to
everyone. (Beat.) Look, I know this isn't
easy...but you're handling this very well.

                    EVELYN
I guess so.

                    JULIA
They say that when you have something to
look forward to, it shortens recovery
time. That's why this new community would
be great for you.

                    EVELYN
Oh, I don't know. I have forty years of
memories in that house. Your father...he
made us a wonderful home.

                    JULIA
Please don't use the words "wonderful" and
"father" in the same sentence.

                    EVELYN
(Beat.) I think it's time we talk about
your father. We pretend like it never
happened.

                    JULIA
When you get out of surgery, I'll take you
over to Orchard Hills. Oh, and here, I
brought some information for you.

Julia shows Evelyn the brochures.

                    EVELYN
Julia, I tried to do my best...but things

were complicated. I was young and I/
didn't...

                    JULIA
/Look, they have tennis courts, a
community rec room, and look at these
beautiful trails. It'll be no time when
you're walking, even running again.

                    EVELYN
We had a good life, even if things in the
beginning were bad.

Julia's BlackBerry rings. She picks up.

                    JULIA
Julia Larson. (Beat.) Yes Edward, I spoke
to him. Did you get my e-mail? Did you get
a hold of the arresting officers? (Beat.)
When you do, find out what you can about Mr.
Samuel's condition during his interview?
And, I want an order requiring the
defendant to submit to an examination with
our psychiatrist immediately. (Beat.) I'll
call you when my mom's in surgery. They'll
taking her into the OR soon.

                    EVELYN
How did he kill his wife and child again?

                    JULIA
Mr. Samuels? Bullets to the head.

                    EVELYN
Was he justified in killing them?

                    JULIA
Killing is *never* justifiable.

                    EVELYN
But what if there were circumstances that
led him to do it?

                    JULIA
Each case is different, but in this case it
was cold blooded murder. (Beat.) Mom, we
shouldn't be talking about this. It's too
upsetting. You should rest.

                    EVELYN
Your father...he did bad things.

                    JULIA
Mom. I don't want to talk about Dad.

                    EVELYN
We can't ignore the past. You have to know
I tried my best.

Julia's BlackBerry rings again.

               EVELYN (CONT'D)
TURN THAT THING OFF, JULIA! I'm trying to
talk to you.

                          JULIA
But this could be something important.

Julia looks at her mom, then reluctantly turns
off her device.

                      JULIA (CONT'D)
Are you happy? Now we can have our goodbye
conversation in peace. (Pause.) I'm sorry,
Mom. I didn't mean to...

                          EVELYN
I want you to tell me the things you've
been afraid to say to me about your father.
                    (Closing her eyes.)
I'm ready.

                          JULIA
Why are you doing this? We've *never* talked
about this before.

                          EVELYN
I don't want you to regret not saying what
you wanted to say to me while I was alive.

                          JULIA
I really wish you'd stop talking like
this.

                          EVELYN
There were so many things I wanted to tell
my mother before she passed.

                    JULIA
You're going to be fine, Mom.

                   EVELYN
I don't want to die without knowing how you
feel. I want to know.

                    JULIA
                  (Fed up)
Okay...you really want to know? In the
thirteen years that he was my father, I
don't remember you doing a damn thing to
stop him. There. It's out there. Are you
happy? I said it.

                   EVELYN
I tried to stop him, you have to believe
me.

                    JULIA
He hit me with the metal tube of a vacuum
cleaner and fractured my arm. I wore a cast
for almost three months.

                   EVELYN
He didn't mean to hurt you like that.

                    JULIA
Do you know what happens when an another
animal threatens a cub? The mother
bear...she goes into a fit of rage. She'll
do anything to protect her child.

                    EVELYN
I didn't know what to do.

                    JULIA
We could have left. We could have started a
new life.

                    EVELYN
Left? To where? Where would we go?

                    JULIA
We could have lived with Grandma Kate.

                    EVELYN
I couldn't burden her. She was struggling
back then.

                    JULIA
She would have helped us if she knew.

                    EVELYN
I was too ashamed and I thought things
would get better. You turned out so
well—despite what happened. You're
beautiful...and successful...and strong.

                    JULIA
No mom, I'm not strong. I throw myself into
work. I haven't had a relationship in ten
years. The thought terrifies me. You want
me to date, to meet a man. For what? The
law is the only institution that I trust
and even the law lets me down sometimes. I

tried to run away. Did you know that? The night of that fight in the kitchen, when he tried to make you drink the dirty mop water you accidently spilled. But I got as far as Ginny's house, and I realized that I couldn't leave you. Not with him. So instead, every night, I prayed that he would die. And it was the only good thing that man ever did in his life!

Pause. Evelyn is tired. The sedatives are finally kicking in.

                    EVELYN
You're right. I needed to stop him. I'm so sorry.

                    JULIA
I shouldn't have gotten worked up. I'm sorry. I'm under a lot of pressure from this case. Everyone—even the mayor—has an opinion about it.

                    EVELYN
What's going to happen with your case?

                    JULIA
I don't know, this new development has complicated things.

                    EVELYN
The man...did he have a reason to kill them?

JULIA

He went into a fit of rage after his wife
went on a shopping spree.

EVELYN

There's always a reason. I don't regret
the years that we spent with your dad. It's
made us who we are. It's made you a good
prosecutor.

JULIA

Look, Mom, it's in the past. We need to
focus on getting you better.

EVELYN

I'm not afraid to die, Julia. Not now
anyway.

JULIA

You're not going to die. We're going you
a nice place at Orchard Hills. Maybe
something overlooking the golf course.

EVELYN

Those Old fogeys like to play golf with
their sons, don't they? If I agree to it,
will you agree to...

JULIA

You know I prefer the courtroom to the
bedroom.

Evelyn looks at her.

                    JULIA (CONT'D)
It's a phrase, Mom.

                    EVELYN
You need to interact with humans in a
normal way...not just in a courtroom or on
your typing machine.

                    JULIA
It's called a *BlackBerry.*

                    EVELYN
I think dying will be very peaceful. Even
beautiful. That's what people say anyway.
You just let go.

                    JULIA
Mom, don't talk like that.

                    EVELYN
I did the right things in life. I'm sure of
it now.

                    JULIA
Well at least you won't be seeing Dad in
the afterlife. He'd most certainly be in
hell.

                    EVELYN
                    (Quietly)
You never know how God judges acts of
honor.

                    JULIA
What did you say?

                    EVELYN
I'm tired.

Julia tucks Evelyn in.

                    JULIA
You should get some sleep. Promise me that
we'll look at Orchard Hills once you're
back on your feet.

Evelyn shakes her head. She starts to nod off,
and gets less cohesive.

                 JULIA (CONT'D)
You'll be running around in no time.

                    EVELYN
Oh good, Julia. I gotta be quick to outrun
Arthur.

                    JULIA
Why do you have to outrun dad?

                    EVELYN
He was heartless, but it wasn't his heart.

                    JULIA
Mom, what are you talking about?

                    EVELYN
                  (Mumbling)
     He didn't die of a heart attack.

                    JULIA
     What are you saying, Mom? What did dad die
     of then?

     Evelyn is passed out. JULIA shakes her mother
     to wake her up.

                    JULIA
     Mom! What did he die of?

          LIGHTS OUT. END OF PLAY.

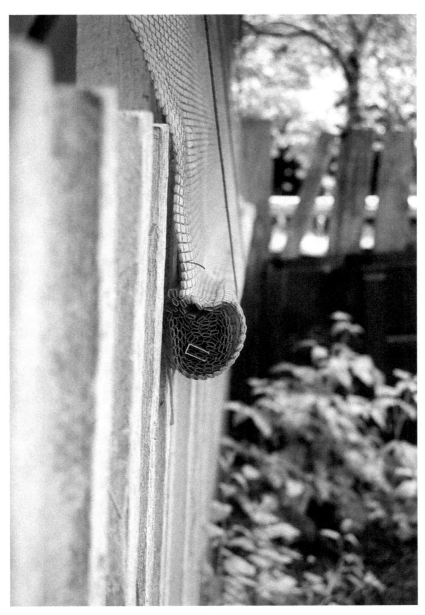

LOST IN TIME
Photograph by Dee Moore

THE END WAS NEAR

Poem by Matthew J. Spireng

I was talking on a cell phone and walking
the dog on the shoulder of the road when
I suddenly realized the end was near. A deer

was about to jump over the guide rail
on the opposite side of the road as a
pickup truck was approaching fast

on my side. It was clear the deer
would leap onto the road and either
the truck would swerve and hit me

and the dog or hit the deer, which
would be thrown into me and the dog,
and then careen into me and the dog

as well. *Hold on! Hold on!* I said
into the cell phone, and then the deer
turned and disappeared down the embankment

on the opposite side of the road and
the truck sped past and I was left
to resume the conversation

knowing how in an instant—
that one, or another—everything
might change.

A FEW FREAK THINGS

Nonfiction by Nyla McCarthy

"We would rather be just like us—and have that be all right."
—Barbara Kingsolver, *The Poisonwood Bible*

I experienced a week in a coma. Underwent two brain surgeries. Relearned how to walk and talk.

This took place in 1967, right after my twelfth birthday.

Gifted the dubious honor of riding out my grandmother's 17 hand Standardbred gelding, Sultan, I was afraid of disappointing her. He was too much horse for me. I was only a fledging rider. I knew it. I rode anyway. So, yeah.

Freak accident. One of those things. Hoof to the head. Lights out.

Once I emerged from my coma and negotiated the basics sufficient to satisfy a team of neurosurgeons, they gauged me ready to go. Then they banished me to Special Education in my soon-to-be junior high.

The term was well underway when I was taken in hand, led from classroom to classroom by Mrs. Christensen, school counselor. Driven by some misguided fuck-fest of good intentions, she stood me up before each and every classroom to make an introduction.

"Class, this is Nyla. Nyla has suffered a terrible accident. She will be joining us at Cascade Junior High School. I know you will all be nice to her. Does anyone have any questions?"

She'd scan the classroom while I faced the inevitable looks of horror that followed when people took in the shiny, synthetic ash-blond wig sitting atop the army-green, fiberglass helmet I was forced to wear to protect my shattered skull.

I'd focus upon nothing while fashionably clad daughters studied the big-headed freak before them dressed in a gold mohair hand-me-down Empire dress and shiny black K-Mart plastic shoes.

The dress was a gift from my Aunt Linda. While two seasons old, I thought it pretty. I forced a smile, ignoring the wave of snide titters, side comments, and judgmental expressions breaking out on the cool girl's faces.

There were never any questions.

I died a thousand deaths, classroom by classroom, that day. Believed I couldn't suffer any fate worse than that humiliation, until Mrs. Christiansen pushed me into one final classroom, away in the darkened corner of the very back of our school.

No introductions were made here. She spoke a few quiet words to the teacher, gestured to a desk, and said, "Miss Jeanette will take it from here."

She walked out the door, leaving me to my fate.

Until this turn of events, I'd survived by adopting a role: *Long Suffering, Proud Survivor*. Within a heartbeat, I recognized this role wasn't going to cut it.

I sat, stunned. Transfixed.

It's important to understand that special education in those days was nothing more than warehousing. No specialized curriculum. No person-centered planning. No Individualized Education Plans. No hope.

The expectations were low. A Special Education teacher's job was mainly to babysit. Keep us safe from one another. Provide us the occupation afforded by whichever games or toys might be available. Keep us quiet.

Miss Jeanette's classroom was decorated with bright posters in the limited palette of primary colors one finds in kindergarten classrooms: dancing ABCs, a simple barnyard bestiary, Dick and Jane doing whatever the hell it is Dick and Jane do.

A single fat, tri-colored hamster circled, listless: a brown-white-reddish blur upon the wheel within a clear, glass tank in the corner. The room smelled of bleach.

A couple of my new classmates studied me with interest. One girl, face marked by a hideous purple scar in the shape of a clothing iron, stem vents and all, smiled. Warm.

An exceedingly thin boy sitting next to her met my eyes, glanced away. Nervous. His head was close-shaved. I realized he had only two fingers on each hand. He was wearing something resembling a judo outfit, though at this time in my life, I had no idea what judo was.

The boy darted another glance at me, returned to drawing on the piece of paper he held in place with one of his unique hands. In the other, he gripped a black jumbo felt pen, sketching a detailed house. His trees were quite realistic, branches and leaves spilling to the ground.

A tiny girl with Down Syndrome (another thing I had no label for) laughed with delight—probably at my helmet, since she couldn't take her eyes away from my oversized, bilious green and blonde head. She began singing "Mary Had a Little Lamb," her thin, sweet soprano rising toward the lights, the sight of my head absorbed, then forgotten.

Off in the corner, separate from everybody else, a disheveled boy with shaggy, unevenly cut hair sat rocking, his hand deep within his pants. He glared at me, a powerful evil eye, muttered, "Go kiss your sister. Go kiss your sister," then laughed. A nasty laugh.

I turned from him toward the teacher.

Miss Jeanette was young, no more than 24. She smiled, kind, but even I could tell she was in over her head. She handed me a plastic puzzle featuring red, blue, green, and yellow, geometric shapes. Suggested in her saccharine, high-pitched girly voice—an infantilized woman's voice I have come to loathe—that I might want to put it together.

I fought back tears, turned to smile at the friendly girl with the iron-shaped scar.

Her name, she told me, was Megan. Though the popular kids made fun of her and called her "Maggot."

"It seems," she shared, "that there are nicknames for everyone in Special Ed."

I was soon to learn my own.

I stared at the puzzle with contempt. Contemplated my future.

Perfect Student was not going to help me on this island of misfit toys to which we had all been banished. *Long Suffering, Proud Survivor* likewise held no promise. I needed to figure out a new identity. Some kind of strategy. Fast.

The next morning, as I stood bare-headed before the bathroom mirror studying my pulsing brain, visible behind the thin skin which covered, but didn't protect it, a realization struck me in a cosmic flash: I would survive best by serving.

When Rodney, the boy busy rocking, told me again to go kiss my sister (a sign, I learned years later in my work with Intellectual/Developmentally Disabled individuals, of severe sexual abuse), or Lance, the two fingered artist, hummed a pitch perfect rendition of the theme song from *Valley of the Dolls*, while the two girls, Megan and Candace, erected domino train after domino train to knock down, I further considered my moment of inspiration.

I needed to learn everything possible about my peers and find appropriate ways to support them. My service identity demanded active advocacy for my disabled sisters and brothers. I could not yet imagine, or explain, what such advocacy might look like.

I took a deep breath, filled myself with outward good cheer and morphed into the *Person Who Triumphs Over the Odds*.

First, to learn about my peers…

Rodney lived in a group home. His father died in Vietnam, leaving his mother alone with Rodney and a little sister. His mother's live-in boyfriend enjoyed making Rodney kiss, and more, his sister. He sodomized both children whenever mom was at work. When she discovered them naked one day, performing as directed, all hell broke loose. The sister was allowed to remain at home. Rodney was carted off to a treatment facility, which, from what I could see in Miss Jeanette's classroom, hadn't been successful. The boyfriend disappeared.

Rodney shared his story with me through fits and starts over a period of weeks, muddled facts mixed with emotion. His cognition was greater than he let most people know. He rocked and rocked, fondled himself, shouted out in defiance, "Go kiss your sister," but for some reason, graced me with rare moments of candor while sharing his harrowing truth.

Lance, I discovered, was a musical and artistic prodigy. A Thalidomide baby born with two fingers on each hand, Lance had been gifted the ability to play xylophone as proficiently as a concert master. He could hear a song once, then play it by ear—perfectly—while gripping long, heavy percussion mallets between his two fingers.

Lance was shy, socially awkward, and sweet. His sister, Jana, a math whiz in the "mainstream" classes, filled in the details for me when we ended up becoming friends.

Megan… oh, Megan, my heart weeps at your memory.

Megan's family died when Megan was quite young, sometime before first grade. Having no known relatives, she became a ward of the state. Placed in one foster home after another, Megan was beaten, raped, chained to a table in a darkened room, all before the age of 10.

At 11, she was placed with a "good" family of a Southern Baptist Elder and his wife, who took in displaced children as casually as some people take in stray cats.

Megan was assigned household chores: dishes, vacuuming the entire house, washing the family's laundry, ironing, folding it.

One Saturday, while watching forbidden cartoons in the rarely empty house, Megan left the hot Rowenta iron a few seconds too long on one of the Elder's dress shirts. A small section of sleeve scorched pale yellow before she noticed. When the family returned, discovered what had happened, the mother slammed Megan down against the kitchen table while that Elder placed the steaming iron against her cheek. He held it there until her flesh melted.

Megan shared this story with me one afternoon as she sneaked a forbidden smoke in the girl's bathroom. She remained affectless throughout the telling. However, her eyes met mine in silent pleading when a couple of girls came in, noticed us huddled together talking, called us "lezzies," and snarled, "You're not supposed to be smoking in here, Maggot."

Candace was the only other one within our "special" caste who came from a regular family. She had one brother, a sister, and two parents who loved her. Candace arrived at school each morning smelling of Ivory

Soap and dressed in colorful gingham or floral little-girl dresses, her ubiquitous bowl haircut neatly combed.

Candace loved to sing. Her cheerful voice could be heard throughout the day singing nursery rhymes or fragments of television advertising jingles. She was blessed with a small, clear, lovely soprano.

We became close, this little band of outsiders.

Sharing our stories. Helping one another practice saying, then doing, socially correct things. We practiced so that when we exited the security of our classroom, we'd fly under the radar. Of course, since each of us stuck out—the proverbial sore thumbs—we never did.

I might come upon Lance in a hallway, being egged on by a group of jocks to "make the vacuum cleaner noise," which he could mimic to perfection. Or they'd be coaxing him to sing nasty lyrics, which he didn't understand, but which were certain to get him into trouble.

Megan was often surrounded by a small trio or dyad of mean girls, taunting "Maggot" as they demanded to know why she smelled so bad. She didn't.

Candace, they pretty much left alone, though that hateful word, "Retard," could be heard, accompanied by snickering, as she made her way, brave and proud, through the halls.

Rodney was often chased around corridors, cornered until he cowered, wetting himself. He'd shout back at his bullies in self-defense, "Go kiss your sister. Go kiss your sister."

Unspeakable cruelty.

Once, I rounded a corner to discover a group of four football players at it. I placed myself physically between them and Rodney, who'd begun shaking, whining something inaudible.

"Stop it!" I erupted. "What in the fuck is wrong with you?! You're supposed to be the good kids."

"Ooooh, Ny-lah," one of them retorted.

"Protecting her boyfriend," another tossed out.

They hooted. Circled us. Began chanting, "Ny-lah. Ny-lah. Rod-ney."

Then caromed away to preen for the popular girls.

I grew fierce, more vocal about the treatment of my special ed family. I wrote a letter to our school newspaper exposing the abuse taking place. I confronted our principal, demanding he make a statement at an assembly. He didn't. I attended a school board meeting, something unusual for a student in those days. I asked to be put on the agenda. After I sat through the entire meeting, they claimed they'd run out of time.

As the year progressed, whenever I walked down the halls, the same boys who harassed Rodney and Lance began to oink at me, make jokes about "Helmet Head Ny-lons," call me *Bald Eagle, Freak Thing*, attempt to yank my wig from my head.

I'd face them in defiance. Then, when I reached home, I'd cry myself to sleep.

Meanwhile, thick black frizz began sprouting across my head.

During my final neurosurgery, they attached a metal plate to my shattered skull, promising that once the ugly, red surgical scars healed, I would no longer need to wear the helmet underneath the wig.

"Your hair will grow back out, Nyla," they reassured, "give it a few months."

But I was done with it all.

When that frizz was barely an inch long, I threw the helmet and the wig into the trashcan, never to be seen again. I looked as butch as most of the women I would later date.

I vowed that I would never let anyone be bullied again if there was anything I could do to prevent it.

It is a vow I have kept. A vow which guides my work.

One black-and-white photo-booth frame survives my emotional purge of all evidence of that horrific period of my life. In it, I am wearing that dull blonde wig, styled in a *de rigueur* Flip hairdo, one side hanging limp despite the barrage of Aqua Net meant to hold it in place. I am wearing my much-mocked mohair dress.

My head is turned slightly to the side in unconscious mimicry of a fashion model's pose.

And my eyes stare, bold and challenging, into the camera.

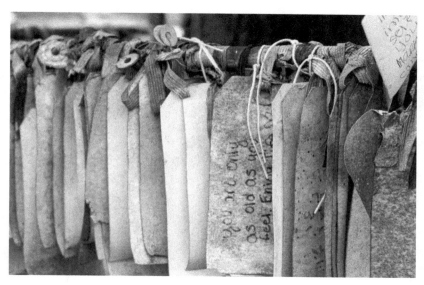

WISHES
Photograph by Micki Selvitella

DRESSED IN WHITE

Fiction by Maddie Silva

There is no one like my mother. She's angelically beautiful. Sun-tanned skin, cerulean eyes, yellow hair. Only ever dressed in white, like a bride or an angel or a snow goddess. White cotton dresses down to her knees, pleated at the skirt and ruffled at the sleeves. She keeps her hair down, falling over her shoulders, long and crimped like strands of crinkle-cut fries.

When I was little, she'd spin me around in our carpeted apartment until the downstairs neighbor thumped at their ceiling with a broom. She'd laugh with her head thrown back, and I'd laugh too, like everything inside me was coming up sun kissed. Even when she set me back down, I'd still feel like I was spinning, her white dress billowing out from under us, her face splitting into rays of joy.

I think about those days a lot now. Just me and her in our little apartment. Just me and her in this large world, living our puny lives. I watch the door of my room constantly, waiting for her white dress to float past the door frame.

Any day now, she'll visit me.

White ceiling, white walls, white floor. White ceiling, white walls, white floor. White sheets, white pillow, white blanket. White sheets, white pillow, white blanket. White ceiling, white walls, white floor. White ceiling, white walls, white floor. White sheets, white pillow, white blanket. White sheets, white pillow, white blanket.

It's been many days since I've arrived here. Maybe even weeks. I've lost count. It's hard to focus on anything in this room with nothing to do and nothing to look at.

It's just me and my stringy thoughts. Those random, terrible thoughts that wriggle their way into my brain and stay there like chewed up and spat out gum. Thoughts like buildings burning and children drowning and men beating their wives and mothers strangling their babies.

I'm not saying I think of these things. These are just the thoughts a person is forced to face when there's nothing else to occupy the mind.

That's why I think about my mother instead. How wonderfully iridescent she is. Sparkling in her dresses, humming to herself around the apartment, picking me up and pointing out the lights in the sky.

There's a man who stands by my room all day. He's fat. He has serious eyes and watches me like I'm about to crawl up the walls and escape through the vent. Maybe he's hungry and wants to kill me for a snack. I try not to look at him, but it's hard not to look back when someone is staring at you.

There's also a lady who comes to my room three times a day. She's bony. She has serious eyes too, and a jaw like a knife. Whenever she comes into the room, she looks at me like I'm wearing someone else's skin to keep warm.

The man watching my room and the lady with a jaw like a knife trade secrets with their eyes when they think I'm not looking. They say all kinds of things with their serious eyes. They don't say anything out loud, but I know what they're saying.

Keep an eye on that girl. She's wearing a child's skin to keep warm.

Last night when I slept or earlier this afternoon when I napped, I dreamt of the play yard where my mother used to take me. All the men who sat by the baseball field were there. They chittered to each other like chipmunks and sang to us while we walked to the jungle gym. The swings creaked in the wind. The wood chips crunched under my feet like ice on teeth.

Wait for me, I was telling my mother in the dream when she let go of my hand and started walking away. Her smile was all lumpy, her eyes all droopy. She wasn't wearing white because that was when her cotton dresses didn't fit anymore. Her belly was growing every day like an alien was trying to get out.

My mother had Monty in our apartment. Birthed her right on the carpet floor. The woman across the hall came to help, but I don't think she did much good. My mother still screamed and screamed until Monty slipped out all bloody and rubbery like a battered toy. The woman across the hall took the bloody towels to the laundry machine and told me to let my mother sleep. I stayed quiet, but my mother didn't ever close her eyes. She spent all night cradling Monty, watching her do nothing.

My mother took out her white dresses again when her belly wasn't so big. After Monty could walk and talk and run and after the playground started filling up with kids from school. When we'd get home, my mother would whirl around, and the dress would fly up like it had before. She'd smile and pick Monty up, spinning her around like a merry-go-round.

I'd watch, nibbling on my nails, waiting for my turn.

Monty came into my dream last night. We were walking down the street to the playground. She was waddling after me trying to keep up. I was pinching her to make her go faster. She cried and cried, but I didn't stop. The crows were glaring at us and trying to herd us off their curbs. I pinched her until we got to the playground. Then I made her sit in the sandbox.

The dream wouldn't move past there. I just kept dreaming about her sitting in the sandbox. Crying until all the sand around her was wet.

Today they brought me a cat in a wire cage. Last week, it was a hamster in a shoebox. The company isn't bad. The cat is black with white paws and big brown eyes. They tell me her name is Mrs. Kittens. They clutch my wrist and show me how to pet her gently even though their grip feels like metal cuffs crushing my bones.

Mrs. Kittens mostly walks around the room, rubbing against the wall and swiping her tail all over the white. She's probably looking for something interesting, but I tell her that she's not going to find it here. I tell her that I've been here for months, and they haven't brought me anything interesting, except for her.

I tell her how much I wish my mother would visit.

I think my days and nights are mixed up. I sleep when the man is watching me, and I'm awake when he's gone. I like it when he's not there because I can think and look around the room without him telling the lady what I'm doing. Except today I keep hearing my mother yelling at me, and I don't think she'd do that if he was there watching.

What's the matter with you?

Her fingers pinch my side. She tells me to sit still, sit alone, be good, be better.

She's sitting in the corner of my room, looking at herself in the mirror, almost perfect now. In her white cotton dress and with her hair almost down to her hips. Her face is empty, blank, and slowly transforming.

I stay where I am because that's where I'm supposed to be. Monty appears by the door.

Don't touch. Be good. Mother's getting ready, I yell at Monty. She watches me with those damp, glossy eyes.

My mother glares at me in the mirror. She reaches for Monty and helps her up on her lap. She decorates Monty's face like she decorates her own, laughing like it's easy. She holds her up and admires her.

When Mrs. Kitten comes back, she curls up next to me now. She doesn't mind the way I pet her. I pet and pet and pet. All her hair sheds onto my pristine sheets. Her throat rumbles against my side. I like the way she feels, and I like the way her little purr fills my empty room.

I tell Mrs. Kittens about my dream last night. How I was watching my mother spin Monty around and around in her white cotton dress. How the pleats billowed up and flew like a saucer. How she had bought Monty a matching dress, so they were like two clouds twirling through space. How I watched and watched until I turned into a boiling pot of water. Then I woke up sweating.

I tell Mrs. Kittens that when I woke up, I couldn't remember what Monty looked like. How odd it was that her face was all blurred out in my mind. Mrs. Kittens purrs. I tell her that it's probably been years since I saw Monty's face.

Maybe when my mother visits, she'll bring Monty, and I'll remember what she looks like.

The lady with the jaw like a knife has her hands on me now. She brings me back to my bed. Her voice whaps me like a stick. *Lie here. Legs up. Don't move. Stay still.*

Something happened. I haven't been in my room for days. I think they've scraped out my stomach or poured acid down my thighs. I hurt so much I sleep for days.

When I wake up, my sheets have turned bright red like the towels my mother gave birth to Monty on. I fall back asleep and wish Mrs. Kittens were purring next to me.

All of my insides are vibrating. I'm sore all over. My hands keep rubbing my belly trying to wipe away the pain. I wish my hands would stop trying to move. Every movement feels like I'm being shoved into the stomach of a house through a mouse hole.

The lady with the jaw like a knife keeps coming into my room and saying things, but I can't understand her gibberish. I wish she would stop talking and leave me alone. Finally, I just close my eyes until she walks away. I can still feel the man by my room staring at me. He's probably wondering where I've been.

I try to fall asleep. I know my mother will visit me when I wake up.

I try to ask the man by my room if my mother has arrived, but I can't get out of bed. My body feels like an anchor at the bottom of the ocean. My white sheets aren't the color of the walls and the floor anymore. They've been rusty all day.

I shout from my bed, but the man doesn't say anything. He just watches me, and the lady comes to watch me too. I ask louder and louder, but words aren't coming out of my mouth. I think I'm just howling.

The dream came back. My mother is spinning Monty around and around and around. Except this time, I don't boil into a pot of steaming water. This time Monty slips from my mother's hands and smashes against the wall like a watermelon. She crumbles into pieces and slumps against the floor. There is a red welt on the back of her head, the size of a cherry pie.

My mother wails for hours like a wolf does to the moon. I frantically try to pick up the pieces. Put them back together. Anything to keep my mother from howling. That's when the woman from across the hall barges in and freezes at the sight. She's struck by lightning, standing there. She looks at my mother, horrified.

I jolt awake when my mother looks to me.

Sitting upright in my bed, my stomach hurts so badly, and my sheets are all wet. I have a terrible, terrible feeling.

Mrs. Kittens came back today. She has something in her mouth. Something big and bulky. She drops it in the corner and jumps up on my bed. She lays by me and purrs.

I squint into the corner. It's a baby, rocking in a diaper and pulling at her feet. I pet Mrs. Kittens and watch the baby. Her babbling fills the room. The baby rights itself, and I see that it's Monty. She smiles at me, smacking her hands against the wall. She's painting the room with every color I know. I watch her all night, smiling until I cry.

When my mother comes to visit, she'll be so pleased to see Monty is here.

The next day, Mrs. Kittens is gone and so is Monty. I must be awake during the day now because the man is there at the window, watching me. The lady with a jaw like a knife is in my room, moving my legs and arms around. Her latex gloves make me recoil. She's telling me things, but I'm not listening. I'm searching the corner for Monty, the walls for the colors.

Have you seen my baby?

Spit flies from my lips. The lady with a jaw life a knife looks at me, valleys etched into her forehead. She looks angry at me for asking. She looks at my skin like I'm wearing someone else's.

Don't you understand anything? The doctor has already seen you for your procedure.

What procedure? I say, but it only comes out mouthed. I look at the man by the door. His eyes are black holes.

Tubal ligation is not reversible.

I shake my head, trying to tell her I don't understand her gibberish. Her jaw like a knife hardens. What she says next, I understand through earthquakes erupting under my stretched and probed skin.

You'll never be a mother.

It must be nighttime. The man by the door is gone. In the corner of the room, there is rustling. I hobble over and see Monty, slumped over like a baby doll. Her lips are dry as tumbleweeds. Worry hangs from her eyebrows like monkeys.

The red welt on the back of her head is still there, smashed in and ringed like a rotted tree trunk. I scoop her up and sit against the white wall. She's cold.

I look at her face, but it is still blurred out. With all my might I try to remember what she looked like before the accident, but this white room makes me forget things.

Like how it feels to spin in my mother's arms. Like how Monty's footsteps sound when she follows me around. Like how long I've been here. Like what my mother told the neighbor that day in the apartment.

Tomorrow our mother will visit, I tell Monty. Tomorrow, she will explain everything.

GAME NIGHT

Script by N. Eleanor Campbell

EXT. FRONT DOOR—NIGHT

PETE(29) raises an arm to knock on the door to
a small home, somewhat overrun by weeds. Holds
a bottle of pricy red wine.

Without knocking, he lowers his fist. Places
the wine on the cheery welcome mat. Turns.
Gingerly starts walking away.

                    JESS
  Where do you think you're going?

JESS (32) stands in the doorway, holding the
wine bottle.

Pete trudges inside the house. Passing her,
snags the wine.

INT. LIVING ROOM—NIGHT

                    MOM
  Peter! You came!

MOM (64) gives Pete a hug and a kiss on the
cheek. She fits the room's décor; it's covered
in cutesy slogans on pillows and childhood
photos of PETE and Jess.

                    PETE
          I said I would, didn't I?

                    JESS
          Let me take your coat.

She glares at him until he hands over the coat
and the wine.

                    BRIT
          Pete, it's been too long. Good to see you
          again.

BRIT (36) in jeans and flannel, offers Pete her
hand to shake.

                    PETE
          You too. You too.

                    BRIT
          Right. Pete makes four. Let's play.

Setting herself back on the couch, Brit bangs a
deck of cards on the coffee table and shuffles.

                    MOM
          Oh! What are we playing?

                    PETE
          Hearts.

Brit stops shuffling. Mom and Brit look at Pete
in surprise.

> PETE (CONT'D)
> What? I do read your emails!

Jess returns with a snack tray, sets it on a side table.

> JESS
> And how are we supposed to know that when you never respond to them?

She sits beside Brit on the couch. Brit puts an arm around her.

> MOM
> Oh, stop pestering your brother, Jess. Shall we play? What are we playing again?

> BRIT
> Hearts.

> PETE
> Which you CAN play with three people. I could just watch or—

> JESS
> Sit down and be happy about it, Pete. You might actually enjoy time with your family for a change.

Jess gives Pete an icy smile.

Brit deals the cards aggressively: in four piles.

Mom's smile is genuine and warm.

                    PETE
    Fine! I'll play.

Pete grabs the pile Brit dealt him and fans
out the cards.

Behind his cards, Pete's frown turns to
concentration. Quick and sharp, Pete
methodically rearranges his cards.

Jess's technique mirrors his. She raises three
cards a centimeter above the others in her
hand. Glances at Pete.

His hand too has three cards poking above the
rest. He gives her a grin. Switches one of the
chosen cards.

Brit sets her three chosen cards down on the
table.

                    MOM
    I have the two!

Mom places the TWO OF CLUBS in the middle of
the table.

                    JESS
    Mom, we have to pass first.

                    MOM
Oh. That's right. Sorry. It's been a while
since we had enough people for Hearts.
Which way do we pass?

                    JESS.
Left.

                    PETE
Left.

                  PETE(CONT'D)
Jinx. You owe me a soda.

                    MOM
I have soda downstairs if you want one,
Dear.

                    JESS
Do you even drink soda?

                    PETE
Of course not! Do you have any idea how
many carbs are—It's just—It's what you
say! Are we going to pass or what?

Jess slides the three raised cards from her
hand to Pete, giving him the evil smile only a
big sister can muster.

He returns the impish grin of a youngest
sibling. Eyes on Jess, he slides cards to Mom.
Picks up the cards from Jess.

                    JESS
Mom, what are you doing? You have to pass
to Brit before you can look at what Pete
passed you.

                    MOM
I do

                    PETE
Yes!

                    MOM
Since when?

                    PETE
Since always!

                    BRIT
Why don't we start a new round?

Brit collects the cards, shuffles, and deals.

                    MOM
Is this some stupid rule your father made
up? Like "No singing?"

                    JESS
Actually, "No singing" is Pete's rule.

                    PETE
You're the one who wouldn't stop singing
show tunes while we were trying to play.

Brit finishes dealing. Everyone picks up their cards.

Jess hums "Seasons of Love."

Pete passes three cards to Mom as he glares at Jess.

> PETE (CONT'D)
> "No humming" is a correlate of "No singing."

> MOM
> Oh! Pete, you passed me the two!

She plays the TWO OF CLUBS.

> JESS
> Mom, I haven't passed yet.

> PETE
> Jesus Christ!

INT. KITCHEN—NIGHT

Pete runs his fingers through his hair. Lets out a deep breath.

Leaning against the wall, Pete slides to the floor, pinching the bridge of his nose, eyes closed.

A hand offers him a glass of red wine.

Pete looks up at Jess standing over him.

He takes the glass. Sips as she slides down next to him. Spits the wine back into the glass.

                    PETE
     That is not what I brought.

                    JESS
     You always bring GOOD wine. I take it home
     and save it for important guests. This is
     the cheap stuff.

                    PETE
     Seriously?

                    JESS
     Drink it. It has a higher alcohol content
     anyway.

                    PETE
     Fair enough.

                    JESS
     Sorry I was humming.

                    PETE
     Sorry I stormed off.

                    JESS
     We better get back. Brit and I only have

the babysitter till ten and you haven't
seen Mom in over a year so you should
probably, you know, actually see her.

She gets to her feet. Offers him a hand. He
accepts.

INT. LIVING ROOM—NIGHT

Cards in hand, everyone sits with exaggerated
politeness.

                    JESS
     Okay. Everyone ready to pass?
     Nods all around.

                  JESS (CONT'D)
     Good. Go ahead.

Everyone passes three cards to the left. Picks
them up and adds the cards to their hands.

                    BRIT
     Who has the two?

Pete checks his hand. The TWO OF CLUBS.
Reaches for it—

                    MOM
     I do!

Mom plays the TWO OF HEARTS.

Pete stares at it. Looks up at Mom in dawning comprehension.

                    JESS
    Mom, that's—

                    PETE
    Jess.

Jess looks over at him. He flicks his head to the door.

INT. KITCHEN—NIGHT

                    PETE
    How long?

                    JESS
    What are you talking about?

                    PETE
    Mom. Since when does she not know how to
    play Hearts?

                    JESS
    Hey! Just because Mom and I aren't freaky
    geniuses like you and Dad doesn't mean
    we're idiots.

                    PETE
    Whoa! That is not—I'm trying to talk about
    Mom.

                    JESS

Mom is fine.

                    PETE

Mom is not fine.

                    JESS

You've been gone, Pete. Maybe you forgot,
Mom is a bit of an airhead compared to you.
Always has been.

                    PETE

Not like this.

                    JESS

She's fine. She just... Just... I mean yeah
there was that time with the car. And the
time—But that was just—She's fine—She has
to be—I have kids, Pete! I can't be here
all the time—I can't—I—

Pete's irritation melts to dismay, hardens
into resolve.

                    PETE

—Jess! Jessica look at me. It's OK. It's
going to be OK. First. We take a deep
breath.

INT. LIVING ROOM—NIGHT

                    PETE (V.O.)

Then we go back in there and we play a

game. And it probably won't be Hearts
but it will be fun. And we will enjoy the
evening whichever way it takes us.

SERIES OF SHOTS:

-Pete and Jess reenter the living room, sit
and smile.

-Mom plays a card, everyone exclaims in good-
natured fun.

-Pete throws his hands up in defeat, smiling.

-Everyone laughs, holding a card stuck to
their forehead.

                    PETE(V.O.)
    And when it gets close to ten, you and Brit
    will go home to the kids.

-Brit and Jess put on their coats.

-Hugs all around.

END SERIES OF SHOTS

EXT. FRONT DOOR—NIGHT

Jess gives Pete another hug.

                    JESS
    But what now, Pete? It's not like

everything is fine just because we made it
through one night.

                    PETE
We'll figure something out. Tomorrow. I'm
not going anywhere.

Pete gives her one last squeeze. Steps back
into the doorway.

Mom leans into Pete, both waving goodnight to
Jess and Brit.

Mom turns back inside. Pete follows, closing
the door.

TALLER NOW

Poem by Tor Lowell

Some days we grow as furious as a fairytale.
Tall stretch marks on bark,
scabbed, bleeding in the sap lines,
prayer: wait: prayer
stop believing, but please *prayer*,
limb-to-limb an embarrassment
of immodesty, the stitching in
our body burst and laid bare.

I am in the after now.
I should love the quiet but I just got it
bending my head down
to see how far away the ground is.

I know I'll get used to it.
I always do, as do you,
the chorus of voices I hear
in your own shot-to-the-sky
screaming, fearing
collision with the sun.

You won't. I didn't.
There's always the stop.
Static breeze, and reorientation
a new relationship with the nearness
of the birds.

One day we won't remember missing
how small we used to be.

SELF-PORTRAIT AS COMFORT FOOD
—MARKET STREET OFFICE, 1997

Poem by Amy Baskin

See the white woman
and   her future boss
or a young female   and an older Asian male.
He   asks her in the interview
Will   she get pregnant soon?
She says no, and gently,   kindly lets him know
his question is   illegal in San Francisco.
Anyway—   it doesn't matter.
She gets the job   that isn't meant for her.
She can tell the truth.
She can tell the truth
about the law   in earnest Japanese.
She can honestly say   she doesn't mind the question,
that she never minds   personal questions
in the workplace   about her womb,
that these questions   don't make her wonder
if her future boss   imagines her
sex life as   a matter of timing:
wash the rice until cloudy   water runs clear.
Nest hen on top with eggs.   *Oyako don*   Mother and Child Bowl.
An easy dish.   A real crowd pleaser.
Watch her bow   as she backs out of
the conference room.   Hear her thank him
for forgiving her   for correcting him.

HERE'S MY HEART

Nonfiction by Anne Gudger

Say "I do" on a sticky August day. With seersucker blue sky and lemon sun. With apple blossom clouds so puffy you could eat them. With family and friends. By a lake where peacocks fan iridescent lapis and jade feathers, and a trumpeting swan will spread its wings when your husband says "I do," when he wraps you in a hug, bends you back and kisses you.

Say "I do" right after you say, "Here's my heart."

Your hummingbird heart that trilled so fast your dad asked if you wanted a valium when he hugged you in the bride's dressing room. You in your strapless watermark taffeta dress. Ankle length even though it's 1983 and bridal dresses are extra like all of fashion is extra. You felt lost in the poofy dresses at the bridal stores with their trains, with their endless layers of fabric and tulle. It was like playing dress-up and you are moons from being the girl who romped around the house in stick-out slips pretending they were tutus.

"No," you told your dad when he held you in his dad arms and asked that valium question. "No. I want to feel it all," you said.

"Half?" he asked.

Before you step into the August sun, your arm laced in your dad's, you'll wish your mom and stepdad were here too. Your mom whose credo, "I'll never speak to your father again," is bigger than this moment.

These are the facts: who is with you and who isn't. Family and friends. Your beautiful sisters: your older sis with her honey eyes and chestnut hair. Your younger sis you've called Snow White with raven hair, fair skin, and cherry red lipstick. Your almost husband's family too—his mom and dad, his sister with her husband and their three girls.

You turn your spotlight on love, on your husband, his electric blue eyes, his cleft chin. Lips framed by moustache and beard. His words: "Here's my heart." Later you'll dig around memory to remember who said it first and later you'll know it doesn't matter.

Love your husband with all five foot two inches of you.

Believe "until death do we part" means when you're a brittle old lady.

Soak love on this memory. Ink it on your marrow. You'll need it.

You're 28.

Pregnant.

Your husband hugs you good-bye in the cool end of day. Winter sky bruising up. The smell of mountain and skiing tucked in the fibers of his russet and moss plaid Pendleton wool jacket—the one you'll keep searching for for months, the one your family will have to remind you was blood soaked and thrown away.

He pulls you close in the parking garage. You've just left your sixth month baby check-up. Six months you've been pregnant with your first, which will be your only with this husband.

He pulls you close. Your ear to his chest to his boom, boom heart. Your lunar baby belly firm against him. The baby knocks a tiny baby part between you.

"Ooh, felt that," he says and presses splayed fingers on your belly, the stretch of his hand against the swish of your swimming boy.

"I wish I were going," you say. You skied with him three weeks before. Doctor approved. But tonight you have a double-size stack of student papers to grade and you are baby tired. Plus you can't zip your ski pants.

"I'll see you late tonight," he says.

"I'll slip in beside you while you sleep your crazy deep sleep," he says.

"You won't even know I was gone."

You want to stop right here. Pry open words and sentences. You want to anchor your feet on one sentence, your hands on the line above, turn your body into a wedge and open this space to the Before. You want to yell at younger you and your husband. Stop! Don't go!

That's not his story.

That's not your story.

Your first husband. The one with Montana sky blue eyes and a dimple and a cleft chin. The one with a large chest and narrow hips. The one who wore a 44 jacket when he wore a jacket. The one who preferred jeans and short-sleeved khaki shirts from JC Penney. The one who sang fake opera and danced with you in the kitchen, dipping you until your shoulder length hair skimmed the linoleum. The one wicked smart who studied the stars, loved hard, laughed easy, and always saw the best in people, even when they weren't their best.

You loved him bigger than the sky. The ocean. You loved him beyond the beyond. The part of you you always held back? You gave him that part too. You showed him your girl traumas: your parents' crazy divorce, Dad's drinking, Mom's depression. You showed him how you'd get stuck in being right, how your stubborn boots were your best boots. And still he loved you. You believed him when he said, "I love you times infinity. And I'll still be crazy in love with you when you're 90 and I'm 99." When you'd cross the street, and he'd catch your hand with, "I don't want anything to happen to you." You believed that too.

Your first husband about whom Nana asked, "How'd you pick such a good one?" because maybe she was a little proud and perplexed since you came from a family of drinkers and divorcers.

You wanted something different. This man with his Midwestern stable feet showed up, and your heart said *Yes, that one.* Your first husband who grew up with the same two parents in the same home his dad built. Your first husband with his bass drum heart, thunder heart.

Your first husband who said, "Let's have a baby!" and one month later you were—snap—pregnant.

Then.

You held him hard in the concrete parking lot.

Kissed him good-bye while winter day turned pewter.

You let him go.

He snaked the mountain road heading for a night of night skiing. Near Enumclaw, Washington, on his way to Crystal Mountain, snow flooded the windshield.

When he hit black ice in a curve like a big C, when his Honda Prelude slipped and spun, when headlights sliced the snow-white dark night, lights from an oncoming car—a station wagon, heavy, heavier with four club-bouncer-sized men inside—when he crashed, the scream of metal and glass, when his seat broke free when his head hit the steering wheel, when he cracked his brain when his heart. Stopped. Dead before the man in the car behind could even open his door. You wondered if he floated over his mangled car and beat-up body and all that blood, his atoms turning, *swoosh*, to light. You wondered if his new self watched the wreck and wondered, *What Now?* Wondered how he was going to hold you without a body.

You were home when he crashed, when his heart cooled. You were refilling your teacup with chamomile. Your body swamped in terror. Every atom quivered in a knowing you didn't want to know as your body turned alabaster marble from your bare toes to your scalp, and you felt something split your heart. You told yourself it was baby hormones. You told yourself it was going to be okay. You forced yourself to breathe even though fear torched all your air.

Everything microscoped to this single frame: a pregnant woman alone in her kitchen, her heart trapped in her collarbones, her hands pressed to her belly as her baby kicked, turned in his private pond.

Oceans of tears. Rage split you. Tears cleaved you. Your first husband died, and you walked around with your insides on your outside. Exposed to the marrow. You were a breathing version of the drawings in Grey's Anatomy: skin peeled, muscles and organs pulsing, bones stitching and unstitching. You bawled monsoon tears, left Kleenex pyramids in your wake, screamed at god and the heavens and everything bigger than you that you could think of.

Your family held you up. Your friends. In time, your widow squad too. They all held you while you sobbed and raged. They held you through the black hole of grief. They held you until your asking "Why me?" turned to "Why not me?" Eventually, you saw the goodness. Your husband never fully left. He'd swoop in and wrap around your collarbones, his non-kiss kiss on your earlobes. You saw him in your son. You oozed gratitude for what he left you with.

You stitched up the hole in your heart with threads of lightning. Well. Not completely. That scar is always there. It throbs sometimes. Twitches. Your scar that reminds you of healing, of gratitude. Your scar that's the source of your superpowers: a deeper love, a wider compassion.

You chose your son. You chose you. And life. You chose love.

In time you said Yes to meeting a friend of a friend.

You changed clothes five, six times before he got there.

You smoked a handful of cigarettes, knowing he didn't want to date a smoker.

He was fun and gentle and oh-so-alive.

You went on that first date. An Italian dinner where you sipped chianti and nibbled spaghetti carbonara, where you laughed when he told you about a sailing trip in bad weather that put the period on a souring relationship, where you played the Whose Family is Crazier game.

You said *goodnight* and locked your front door. Then phoned your younger sister, Janis, the one you called Snow White with her black hair and fair skin. You told her, "He's a no. He's too short."

"What?" She laughed through the phone. "Too short? You're barely five two," she said, and you laughed too.

"Come on," she said. "Don't shut it him out so fast."

Guilt and fear held hands and circled you, taunting. Fear roared its roar so you welded copper around your heart because you knew copper bends easier than steel because you did and didn't want to show him your heart.

He kept coming back.

You kept opening the door.

Love your second husband. This honey of a man who tasted like love and jazz music and the ocean. With his tender heart. With his kindness. With his Always-Making-Room-at-the-Table-ness. With his own father loss that gave him a sensitivity to your ache, to your boy. Your second husband who slipped in your life, who loved you up close, who didn't feel threatened by your first husband. You asked. Because people asked you. "How could I feel jealous?" he said. "He loved you like I do," he said. "And he gave you your son," he said. "I'll always be grateful to him."

Marry your second husband on a sun-soaked July day. Marry him after you say, "Here's my heart." After you say, "It's a little bruised, and here it is."

Marry him on your friend's deck overlooking Puget Sound—a finger of water that points to the ocean. Deep blue water. Sky blue sky. Aquamarine. The in-between of water and sky on the horizon where everything is possible. The flood of northwest green in their yard: emerald grass, maple trees dressed in lettuce green, hostas in the shade, that deep woods green with stripes of white.

Your adorable son, two and a half, with his dimple smile and handful of curls, with his hazel eyes, bouncing in his sailor suit and saddle shoes.

He's all toddler joy. He'll laugh and squeal. He'll play with an oversized beach ball while dipping in and out of family arms.

Forge a family. This second chance at happiness when you thought your happy was all used up. Your first husband will zip in too, curling around your collarbones, tickling your earlobes, giving you goosebumps. He'll swoop in like a hummingbird dive bomb, and you'll feel a deeper blessing that getting married is right. It's what he would want for you. It's what you want for you. Your beautiful boy in one hand, stargazer lilies with their streaks of hot pink in the other. You'll poke your head outside to where your almost second husband and his sister sing a love duet. There's your family: sisters and parents. Your mom and stepdad ("I feel like I have a second chance," your mom said when she told you. "Yes, I'll be there this time."). Your dad. Maybe with a valium in his pocket, but he doesn't offer it.

Just before you step from inside to outside, you'll hear your first husband: *I love you. Now go.*

"How'd you pick such a good one?" Nana asked again. Again, maybe she was a little proud and perplexed. And you laughed. You've said it for years: how grateful you are to marry two sweet men. To marry kindness twice.

"Let's have a baby!" your second husband said and, lucky you, one month later you were—snap—pregnant.

"Promise you'll stay?" you said, your lunar belly pressed against him, worry leaking into your words.

"I'll do my best," he said.

"The million-dollar family," a friend said when you called her to tell her you had a girl. Meaning, you guessed: a boy and a girl. Column A.

Column B. First you thought, I took the long way 'round. And then you grinned because, Yes, you felt lucky. You were giddy to be a wisher on stars. A rubber of Buddha bellies. Lady luck. Lucky you. You were grateful "lucky" still knew your address.

While your second husband adopted your son and gave him everything but his genes, you kept your first husband in your family too. Through stories. Through his family being your family. Through celebrating his birthdays with his favorites—German chocolate cake and cherry coke. Through calling him "Dad Kent" because you wanted your son to know. This silent third parent. At the table. In the car. In the quiet of reading at bedtime.

"He was my dad too," your then four-year-old daughter said one night at dinner, and you nearly choked on a carrot. "But he died."

Two husbands. Two kids. Grow your family like you grow your garden in countless rows. Watering with love. Plucking weeds. Making room for joy and laughter and tears and kitchen table talks. Add extended family, friends, cooking, travel, school, books, beach days, forest days, sports. Plant dreaming and doing. Fertilize with art, music, writing. Life's deliciousness.

Time jump to two kid-in-laws.

Stand and witness another July wedding. Your son this time. Your phenomenal boy who came through the stardust. All man in his grey linen suit. In his galaxy-wide heart with his dimple smile. In his choosing a partner who is fire to his water. Your son who carries his dad's wedding ring in his breast pocket. The ring you gave your first husband 35 years ago. The ring you gave your son last night.

Have the reception at your farm. No swans or salty Puget Sound water. This time a gorgeous hay field with a honey sun. Lights strung around the handmade dance floor. A tree full of family wedding pictures:

grandparents, your daughter-in-law's parents, you with your first husband, you with your now husband. Love lights shining. The air lit with magic.

At Toast Time your husband stands behind the bride and groom, clears his throat, wipes a tear with his knuckle. He is all Thanks.

Then.

"And tonight, I have a double toast," he starts.

The well of tears that float between your top ribs perks up.

"Not all of you know, but Annie was married before I knew her," he says.

Your elbows on the table. Hands to your mouth.

"She was pregnant with Jake when her husband died tragically," he says.

"Jake was two when Annie and I got married," he says.

"When he made me a dad."

Blink, blink tears. Breathe. Your daughter, Maria, sitting next to you slides her hand on your knee to anchor you.

"Then our family grew," he says.

"And we had Maria," he says.

"I'm a lucky guy," he says.

"So, my first toast is to Kent," he says and raises his glass. His upper lip quivers. His voice too.

"To Kent Neuberger," he says.

"Who gave you life."

"We wish you were here."

Let yourself be shot through with love. A love infusion. Skies of love. Oceans of love. Love tsunami. Grateful for it all. The hard parts. The beautiful parts. All the parts.

Here's my heart.

TO BE CONSUMED

Poem by Madronna Holden

The humble carrot,
the flamencoed onion
know what it is to be transformed
into sugar and heat
in intimate dissolution
in the belly of another.

This, the garden tells the gardener
is the root and fruit of love.

This is what it is to be consumed
by the open-mouthed wonder
that seeks its course in us

(This is what it is to live.)

as we all take turns
feeding one another.

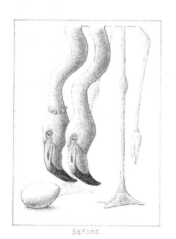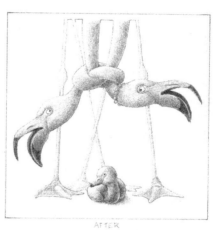

BEFORE AND AFTER
Drawing by C. Lill Ahrens

CONTRIBUTORS

C. LILL AHRENS is an award-winning published author, an editor for *Calyx Journal*, a conference presenter, a retired editorial consultant, and the creator/instructor of The Writers' Ready Room Online, a guided critique class. Many of her students and clients are now award-winning and published. Lill is also an artist so she's drawing a how-to-write book.

CLAIRE ALONGI graduated magna cum laude from Willamette University, where she was the recipient of the Mark and Melody Teppola Prize in Fiction three years in a row. She enjoys writing stories that incorporate the strange and uncanny. You can find her in Davis, California, reading, writing, pestering her cat, watching too many movies, and waiting for indisputable proof that dragons exist.

AMY BASKIN's work is currently featured in Kai Coggin's Wednesday Night Poetry, *Pirene's Fountain*, *Friends Journal*, and is forthcoming in *Pilgrimage*. She is a Pushcart Prize and Best of the Net nominee, an Oregon Literary Arts Fellow, and an Oregon Poetry Association prize winner. When not writing, she helps run literary arts programs including Fir Acres Writing Workshop at Lewis & Clark College.

N. ELEANOR CAMPBELL is a native Portland Screenwriter who seeks truth through fiction by encouraging a second look at assumptions we might hold and by showing examples of heroes we seldom see. Her script "Our Father" made finalist in the 2021 FiLM LaB Competition and her co-written short "Hey, Man" is in post-production. Outside of the writing and film worlds Eleanor works for OHSU as a computational biologist.

MARGARET CHULA has published thirteen collections of poetry including, most recently, *Firefly Lanterns: Twelve Years in Kyoto*. Her poems explore the interconnectedness between our everyday lives and the natural world. A featured speaker and workshop leader at haiku conferences around the world, she has also served as president of the Tanka Society of America, Poet Laureate for Friends of Chamber Music, and is currently on the Advisory Board for the Center for Japanese Studies. While living in Kyoto, she studied the traditional arts of flower arrangement and woodblock printing. Maggie now makes her home in Portland, Oregon.

NATALIE DALE graduated with honors from the Chicago Medical School in 2016 and started residency in Neurology at Oregon Health Sciences University. After struggling with bipolar disorder, she took a leap of faith and left residency to focus on her life-long passion: writing. Since then, her short stories and essays have been published in *Flash Fiction Magazine, Wyldblood, Breath & Shadow, READ White & Blue Anthology*, and the *National Alliance on Mental Illness (NAMI)*, among others. In her spare time, Natalie organizes an elementary school reading program, runs a writing critique group, and plays violin in a community orchestra

CAITLIN CLAIRE DIEHL is the author of the YA fantasy novel, *First Daughter*. Her other book is a fun and practical look at sex and relationships for young women entitled, *Loving Sex: Straight Talk for Straight Girls*. Caitlin has an M.A. in Counseling Psychology. She has a been a member of Willamette Writers and the Northwest Independent Writer's Association. Before focusing on her own writing, she worked as a counselor and college writing instructor. Caitlin and her husband were married 28 years before his death from cancer in 2015.

ANNE GUDGER is an essay/memoir writer who writes hard and loves harder. Previous work can be found at *the Timberline Review, Real*

Simple Magazine, The Rumpus, PANK, Barren Magazine, Winning Writers, Bending Genres, Atticus Review, Sweet Lit, Creative Nonfiction Sunday Short Reads, Columbia Journal, and elsewhere. Plus, she's won three essay contests. She co-founded Coffee and Grief—with her amazing daughter—that includes a monthly reading series because everybody grieves. She lives in Portland with her beloved husband and is lucky to have kids and kid-in-laws not far. More at Annegudger.com, Anne Gudger on IG and fb. Coffee and Grief Community on fb.

MICHAEL HANNER's poetry has appeared in *the Timberline Review, Shark Fish, Gargoyle, Southern Humanities Review, Rhino, Nimrod, Mudfish* and others. His recent books are *October, Adriatica*, and *Le Bugue, Périgord & Beyond*. In 2021 he published *Alice* and *More Alice*, two collections of prose poems about a muse or perhaps someone completely different. His other interests are gardening, travel, English croquet, French cooking, and Argentine tango.

MADRONNA HOLDEN is taking the opportunity of her retirement from university teaching to concentrate on her award-winning poetry, which has recently appeared in over two dozen literary journals, including *The Bitter Oleander, The Cold Mountain Review, Leaping Clear* and *About Place*, and has been selected as poem of the day by *Verse Daily*. The production of her full-length poetry drama, *The Descent of Inanna*, was the subject of a documentary aired on Oregon Public Broadcasting. Her first chapbook is *The Goddess of Glass Mountains* (Finishing Line Press 2021).

LISA S. LEE is a Portland-based writer, speaker, brand and innovation strategist, and entrepreneur. Most of Lisa's writing is grounded in one question: "What does it mean to find one's 'authentic self'?" Her full-length plays include *Chopsticks and Dirty Laundry* and *Girl Against the Wall*, and her 10-minute plays include "The Picnic," "Box of Donuts," and "The Scarf." Her plays have received productions in New York City,

Chicago, San Francisco and Toronto. Her book, *Santa's Boardroom: A Story of How a Company Built a Beloved Brand*, teaches executives and entrepreneurs how to build a brand and lead a brand-led company.

TOR LOWELL is a queer writer and zine-maker. Their previous works have appeared in *Mollyhouse*, *Rhythm & Bones Press*, and *Peculiar: A Queer Literary Journal*, among others. They live in the Pacific Northwest.

KATE MAXWELL has probably been a teacher for way too long. As a result, her interests include film, wine, and sleeping. She's been published and awarded in many Australian and International literary magazines and her first poetry anthology, *Never Good at Maths* is published with Interactive Publications, Brisbane. She can be found at https://kateswritingplace.com/

NYLA McCARTHY lives along the banks of the North Umpqua River where she labors to find, and honor, her voice. A member of the 2021-22 Attic Atheneum Fellowship, she also serves on the board of the Oregon Writers Colony. Nyla is founding chair, now Emerita, of the Portland Commission on Disabilities, past Chair of the Salem Human Rights and Relations Commission, and one of the Creation Committee members for the Portland Office of Equity and Human Rights. Nyla once danced with Big Bird. Really.

DAVID MIHALYOV lives outside of Rochester, NY, with his wife, two daughters, and beagle. His first collection, *A Safe Distance*, will be published by Main Street Rag Press in 2022.

DEE MOORE is a Queer freelance journalist and artist originally from Texas living in the Willamette Valley.

NANCY NOWAK's poetry has appeared in numerous journals and anthologies, including RAIN Magazine. Fireweed, *the Timberline Review,*

Clackamas Literary Review, Jefferson Journal, and *Last Call: The Anthology of Beer, Wine, and Spirits Poetry.* Some of her previously published work can be found at nancynowakpoetry.com. She holds an MFA from Sarah Lawrence College. From 1994 to 2016, she was an associate professor at Umpqua Community College, Roseburg, OR, where she taught writing. She lives in Winston, OR.

KELI OSBORN writes lists, letters, testimony, essays and poems. Her writings have been published in the *San Pedro River Review, Cold Mountain Review, The Fourth River,* and *Confrontation*—and in several anthologies, including *The Book of Donuts* (Terrapin Books) and *All We Can Hold, Poems of Motherhood* (Sage Hill Press). She makes her home in Eugene, Oregon.

KITT PATTEN is a recently retired airline pilot. With her wings clipped, she has come to roost in Tillamook, Oregon. She is delighted to have the time to devote to creative pursuits—writing about real and imagined lives and photographing the amazing world around her. Her writing and photographs can be seen in print in the inaugural issue of *Turbulence and Coffee* and the most recent issue, No. 8, of *The North Coast Squid* literary journal.

JOYCE SCHMID's most recent work appears or is forthcoming in *Five Points, Literary Imagination, Dunes Review, Northwest Review,* and other journals and anthologies. She lives in Palo Alto, California, with her husband of over half a century.

MICKI SELVITELLA is a writer and artist living in the Pacific Northwest.

SANDRA SIEGIENSKI is a speech pathologist living in the Pacific Northwest. Her fiction has placed in the Willamette Writers Kay Snow Writing Contest, the PNWA Literary Contest, and the Romance Writers of America FF&P Contest. Additionally, she has received multiple honorable mentions from the L. Ron Hubbard Writers of the Future Contest. An enthusiastic student of languages, culture, dance, and history, Sandra is currently writing a variety of sci-fi/ fantasy and young adult novels as well as short stories.

MADDIE SILVA is an emerging writer based in Los Angeles. Her writing has appeared in *Loud and Queer Zine* and she is currently working on her first historical fiction novel about the lesbian rights movement during the 60s. Maddie is also an educator for young writers, a runner, a traveler, and a self-proclaimed coffee connoisseur.

MATTHEW J. SPIRENG's 2019 Sinclair Poetry Prize-winning book *Good Work* was published in 2020 by Evening Street Press. An 11-time Pushcart Prize nominee, he is the author of two other full-length poetry books, *What Focus Is* and *Out of Body*, winner of the 2004 Bluestem Poetry Award, and five chapbooks. He was the winner of The MacGuffin's 23rd Annual Poet Hunt Contest in 2018 and the 2015 Common Ground Review poetry contest. Website: matthewjspireng.com.

COLETTE TENNANT has two books of poetry: *Commotion of Wings* and *Eden and After*. Her most recent book, *Religion in The Handmaid's Tale: a Brief Guide*, was published in September 2019 to coincide with Atwood's publication of The Testaments. Her poems have been nominated for the Pushcart Prize and have been published in various journals, including *Prairie Schooner, Rattle, Southern Poetry Review*, and *The Fish Anthology*. She is an English Professor in Salem, Oregon, and curates The Fusion Art Show, featuring student poems, paintings, and photographs.

LUCINDA TREW studied journalism and English at the University of North Carolina at Chapel Hill. Her work has appeared in *The Fredricksburg Literary and Art Review, The Poet, Cathexis Northwest Press, The Bangor Literary Journal, San Pedro River Review, Kakalak, Mockingheart Review, Flying South,* and other journals. She is a recipient of a 2020 Kakalak Poetry Award, a 2019 North Carolina Poetry Society Award, and was named a 2021 North Carolina Poetry Society poet laureate award finalist. She lives and writes in Union County, N.C.

GLEN VECCHIONE is the author of 28 science books for young adults as well as fiction writer and poet. His poetry has appeared in *Missouri Review*, *ZYZZYZA*, *Southern Poetry Review*, *Indiana University Press*, and *Tar River Poetry*. Glen also composes music for television, film, and theatre. Glen currently divides his time between San Diego, California, and New York City.

CRISTINA L. WHITE is a life-long reader, writer, and artist. Her work has appeared in various publications, including *Orion Magazine*, *Willawaw Journal*, *Gay Flash Fiction*, and *Pigeon Review*. Her story "Becoming Art Deco" is due for publication in *Occult Detective* Issue #8, and "One Cup of Rice" is in the anthology *Youth in Wartime*. She is a published and produced playwright, and her film *Tallulah* won the 2021 Local Film Audience Award at the 10th Annual McMinnville Short Film Festival. She writes, makes art, and tends a small garden in Corvallis, Oregon. Find her at cristinalwhite.com.

MELODY WILSON's recent work appears in *Quartet, Briar Cliff Review, The Shore, Whale Road Review, the Timberline Review, SWWIM*, and. She received the 2021 Kay Snow Award, Honorable Mention for the 2021 Oberon Poetry Award, and finalist in the 2021 Patricia Dobler Poetry Award.

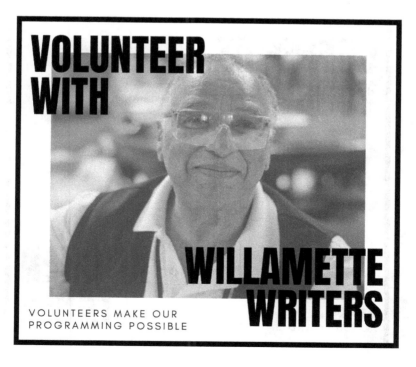

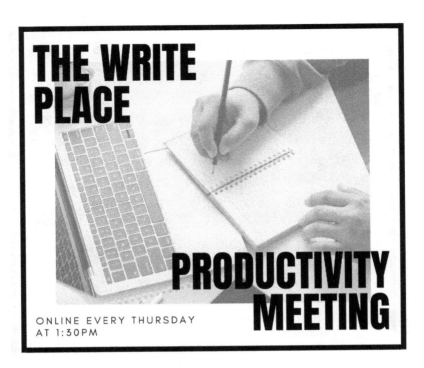

THE WRITE PLACE

PRODUCTIVITY MEETING

ONLINE EVERY THURSDAY AT 1:30PM

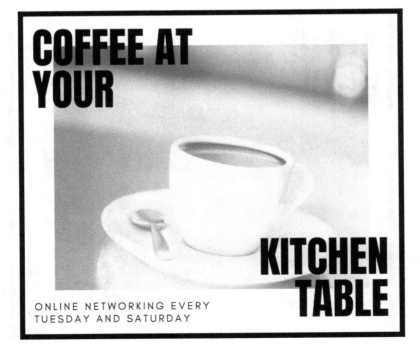

COFFEE AT YOUR

KITCHEN TABLE

ONLINE NETWORKING EVERY TUESDAY AND SATURDAY

CPSIA information can be obtained
at www.ICGtesting.com
Printed in the USA
JSHW042340150722
28134JS00002B/6